# Optimum Nutrition
# for Babies and
# Young Children

# WITHDRAWN

# About the Author

LUCY BURNEY is a qualified Nutrition Consultant and children's health specialist. She trained at the renowned Institute for Optimum Nutrition and then went on to practice at the Hale Clinic, London. She is the author of three books on children's health and regularly contributes to radio and television interviews on the subject. Lucy lives in Berkshire with her husband and their four young children and can be contacted through her website **www.lucyburney.co.uk**

Dear Reader

I hope you and your family find this book helpful. I also hope that when you finish reading it you are sure of the value of improving and maintaining optimum health for your children.

Each child is different, each family works differently and people have different priorities so I have set up a website at

**www.lucyburney.co.uk**

to provide up-to-date information and, more importantly, a place where parents can talk to each other and to me about particular concerns and issues.

Please visit and register and I look forward to meeting you there.

# Optimum Nutrition for Babies and Young Children

**Over 150 quick and tempting recipes for the best start in life**

## Lucy Burney

**PIATKUS**

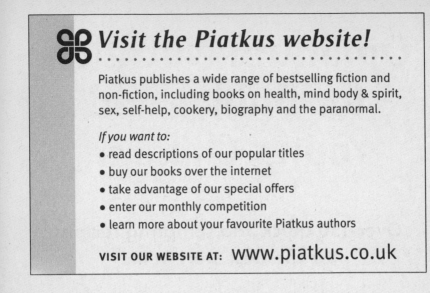

# Visit the Piatkus website!

Piatkus publishes a wide range of bestselling fiction and non-fiction, including books on health, mind body & spirit, sex, self-help, cookery, biography and the paranormal.

*If you want to:*
- read descriptions of our popular titles
- buy our books over the internet
- take advantage of our special offers
- enter our monthly competition
- learn more about your favourite Piatkus authors

**VISIT OUR WEBSITE AT: www.piatkus.co.uk**

© 1999 Lucy Burney

First published in 1999 by
Piatkus Books Ltd
5 Windmill Street
London W1T 2JA

This edition published 2005
Reprinted 2006

e-mail: info@piatkus.co.uk

The moral rights of the author have been asserted

*A catalogue record for this book is available from the British Library*

ISBN 0-7499-2622-8

Design and typesetting by Paul Saunders
Illustrations by Brigitte McDonald

This book has been printed on paper manufactured
with respect for the environment using wood from
managed sustainable resources

Data manipulation by Phoenix Photosetting, Chatham, Kent
Printed and bound in Denmark by Nørhaven Paperback A/S, Viborg

*To Max, Otto (and our newborn, India)*

# Contents

# Acknowledgements

I WOULD LIKE TO THANK some special people without whom this book would not have been written. Many thanks to my agent Laura Morris for her unfailing optimism and belief; to Dr George Lewith for his regular support and knowledge; to Gill and Rachel at Piatkus for their encouragement and guidance; to Michele Duval for helping to care for our boys whilst I was writing and for bringing so much love and laughter into our house. Many thanks to Theresa Laflin, who meticulously tested all the recipes on her family and friends. Finally, to my husband Nigel, who helped me find the confidence I needed and without whom I would never have started writing. My love – thank you.

---

## Author's note

The material in this book is for information purposes only. It is not intended as an alternative to medical advice. If you suspect that your child is suffering from a medical condition, you should always consult a doctor.

I have found myself referring to 'he' throughout the book. This is because, as a mother of two boys, it came more naturally. However, it is meant to refer to children of both sexes.

# Foreword

LUCY BURNEY HAS a wonderful, comprehensive and very practical grasp of the problems involved in clinical nutrition. This professional expertise, combined with her knowledge and experience as a mother shines through and has resulted in a book of great clarity. The recipes are mouthwatering and the text is a paragon of practical common sense and good research.

Clinical nutrition has become increasingly important and relevant over the last decade. We are slowly beginning to realise that some of the food pushed at us from advertising hoardings and television screens is simply not very good for us. In the West we are seeing the rise and rise of obesity. Unfortunately obesity is not based on good healthy eating, but rather on empty calories, sub-nutrition and a lack of exercise. Fats and 'quick fixes' from sweets and chocolate merely put weight on without providing us with the trace elements and vitamins we require. The message that sub-nutrition is widespread and probably an important cause of illness is starting to take root in conventional medicine and my guess is that it will become an increasingly important part of our medical practice over the next two decades.

If our children are going to get the most from life then they have got to remain fit and well for as long as possible. This book introduces a very practical and simple approach to healthy eating. It is vital that we begin this process as soon as we start feeding our children and we should encourage them to have a positive and sensible nutritional outlook. I hope those who read this book will be inspired by Lucy's integrity, enthusiasm and knowledge. And I hope it will make them think twice before giving their child a biscuit or a packet of crisps just to keep them quiet!

Sound nutrition is undoubtedly one of the essential corner stones of a healthy, long and productive life.

Dr George Lewith MA DM FRCP MRCGP

# Introduction

WHAT YOU CHOOSE to feed your child during the first few years of his life will directly affect not only his growth, but also his energy levels, his mood, his resistance to disease and his ability to concentrate and do well at school. I discovered this whilst I was still training as a nutritionist and I was shocked that the information I was researching was not common knowledge. It was then that I made up my mind to write a book on the subject, in an attempt to fill the gaps in the sparse information available.

## How to use this book

In this book I have tried to dispel some of the common myths that surround feeding babies and children up to the age of five. In my opinion it is the first five years that are the most important in terms of a child's diet. This is a time of massive growth and development, and a time when over half your child's learning pathways are formed in his brain. These pre-school years are also the time when, as parents, you have the most influence over your child's eating habits.

I have made the book as user-friendly as possible. Chapter 1 deals with general issues such as food allergies and labelling. After that, each age group has its own chapter with the recipes included at the end. I have also made the recipes as straightforward as possible and often use terms such as 'a handful' or 'a cup' or '1 carrot', rather than specific quantities. If you are a busy mum, you just don't have time to get the weighing scales out every time you start cooking. The beauty of these recipes is that they will not spoil if, for example, you use a large carrot instead of a medium one. Cooking should not be an exact science. Enjoy experimenting with the recipes and adapting them to your own needs. Every family's appetite varies so all the recipes can be halved or doubled very easily.

## Getting the right balance

No child, or parent, for that matter, will eat healthily 100 per cent of the time. During the first two years of your baby's life you can always dictate what is on the menu, but after this time – with the advent of nursery school, tea parties and 'drop offs' – it becomes less easy. I think it is important to have a healthy attitude towards food as a parent. After all, food is one of our greatest pleasures, as well as being our main energy source. If your children are eating healthily 80 per cent of the time, you're doing fine. It is unlikely that the other 20 per cent will adversely affect them. Teaching your children about food will also reduce the risk of mutiny during these early years. Cooking with them and chatting about health gets them interested at an early age. Many of the recipes in the family meals section can be cooked with your children. I also believe in children making their own choices from an early age. Allowing them the freedom to choose what they eat when they are away from home is yet another part of growing up that is fun and should be encouraged. It should also help to ensure that they go on making wise dietary choices as adults.

I have the greatest pleasure in passing on the knowledge I have gained over the years, and hope that you and your family will benefit from it as much as my own and many others have.

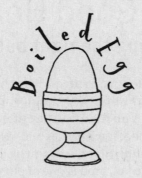

# 1.

# Sowing the Seeds of Good Health

This chapter covers the basic principles of good nutrition as well as a number of general issues concerning healthy eating. For ease of reference, the topics are as follows:

## 'Children's diseases are parents' mistakes'
### HERBERT E. SHELTON

As PARENTS, WE ALL want to do the very best we can for our children. So it is rather alarming that, in spite of modern medicine, our children are becoming more susceptible to disease as each year goes by. As many as one in four children under eight now suffer from eczema, over 1.5 million children suffer from asthma, and up to one in six suffer from allergies. Hyperactivity is escalating out of control, ear infections are now considered a routine part of childhood, and regular visits to the doctor a necessity.

There are certainly many contributing factors. Environmental pollution plays a part, as does genetics. However, without doubt, one of the major causes of childhood illness is diet. Our children's diet has become filled with over-processed, highly refined foods which are too high in salt and sugar, and lack the nutrients required for optimal growth and development. A government survey carried out in 1995 revealed that one in eight children between the ages of 18 months and two and a half years are anaemic (iron-deficient). Iron is an important mineral and a deficiency can cause symptoms of fatigue and listlessness, slow development and frequent colds and infections.

The survey also revealed that, amongst the under-fives, biscuits, white bread, non-diet soft drinks and savoury snacks, along with chips and sweets, were the most commonly eaten foods, consumed by more than 70 per cent of the children. Only half the children ate any fruit at all, and peas and carrots were the only cooked vegetables (excluding potatoes) eaten by more than half of the children. Tea was consumed by a third of the children and those drinking non-diet soft drinks were estimated to be drinking 1.5 litres (2½ pints) per week. It is not surprising therefore to find that pre-school children are failing to receive even the basic recommended levels of many vitamins and minerals.

Without enough of these essential nutrients, children start to develop deficiency symptoms. A child with constipation may be lacking in magnesium or vitamin C. Dry skin and pimples can both be symptoms of essential fatty acid deficiency or lack of vitamins A and C. A poor appetite can be a symptom of an iron or zinc deficiency. Tiredness can indicate that your child is not getting enough of the B vitamins, iron or magnesium.

More importantly, a consistently poor diet in childhood can also affect not only your child's current health, but also his long-term health, increasing the risk of degenerative disease in later life. Research has shown that babies born with a low birth-weight, or who are at a low weight by the age of one, have a much higher risk of developing heart disease and diabetes in later life. Also, some teenage girls are showing early signs of osteoporosis as a result of eating a junk food diet throughout their early years.

## Prevention is better than cure

A child's diet needs to contain unadulterated, nutrient-rich foods: fresh vegetables and fruit (organic wherever possible), whole grains, lean meats, fish (especially oily ones), pulses, dried fruits, ground nuts, seeds and their oils. Children need water and diluted fresh fruit juices to drink, not fizzy drinks or squashes which are full of sugar, colours, artificial sweeteners and stimulants like caffeine. A healthy immune system comes from a healthy diet and, with over 3500 chemicals now being added to our food, we must arm our children with an immune system that can cope with this daily bombardment.

Young children will always get ill; an immune system is built up through exposure to bacteria and viruses. However, with the right approach, using diet and the simple guidelines set out in this book, colds and infections can be dealt with naturally instead of reaching for a doctor's prescription. A child's body has the most marvellous capacity for self-healing if it is given the right nourishment and care. Whatever your child's age, it is never too late to start them on the road to health. Feeding them a fresh, wholesome and varied diet is a gift that lasts a lifetime.

# The building blocks of health

Your child's body is entirely built and maintained by the food he eats, the water he drinks and the air he breathes. In order for his body to function, there are seven main nutritional elements which constitute the building blocks of health: protein, fat, carbohydrate, fibre, water, vitamins and minerals.

## Protein

Protein is vital for the growth and repair of all cells. It can also be used for energy production, if needed, or stored as fat. Protein is made out of 22 amino acids, and the quality of the protein is determined by which amino acids it contains. Eight out of the 22 amino acids are essential, which means we have to get them from the food we eat. The remaining ones are called non-essential, because they can be made from the pool of other amino acids that we store in our bodies.

Surprisingly, your children need much less protein a day than you might think. Babies being breast-fed only receive 1.5 per cent of their total calories from protein, yet they still manage to double their birthweight in the first six months. In the West, both as children and adults, we tend to eat too much protein, rather than too little, which can cause excess acidity in the body and lead to illness.

Good sources of protein are eggs, pulses (especially soya beans and products made from them, like soya milk and tofu), lean meat, fish, cheese, yogurt, nuts and seeds, and certain grains like quinoa. Quinoa is a South American grain, which contains protein of a much better quality than meat.

## SUMMARY

**1.** Give your child 3–5 servings of protein a day. Serve a concentrated form of protein, like meat or eggs, only once a day. These foods can be difficult to digest and are high in saturated fat.

**2.** Include a variety of grain and pulse dishes for additional protein intake (see the vegetarian recipes throughout this book). Look at the menu on page 23 as an example.

# Fat

Fat is a necessary component of our bodies. It keeps us warm, is a source of energy, keeps our skin and arteries supple, cushions our internal organs and is essential for proper brain function. Babies and young children need a higher proportion of fat than adults. However, there are two main types of fat and it is important to distinguish between them because they affect our bodies in very different ways.

The first type is saturated fat – the unhealthy fat which is mainly found in meat and dairy products, including butter, cheese, meat fat and eggs. It is neither desirable nor sensible to include too much saturated fat in your child's diet. Saturated fat is associated with a higher risk of heart disease and inflammatory conditions like asthma, eczema and arthritis.

A much better form of fat to include in your child's diet is unsaturated fat. Unsaturated fat is the healthy fat and is divided into a further two groups: monounsaturated fat and polyunsaturated fat. 'Mono' and 'poly' simply refer to the chemical composition of the fat. Olive oil is an excellent source of mono-unsaturated fat and is by far the best cooking oil because, due to its chemical composition, it is stable at high temperatures. (Polyunsaturated oils, like sunflower or safflower oils, are unstable at high temperatures. This damages them and creates dangerous compounds called free radicals, which have been implicated as a contributory factor in heart disease and cancer.) It is best to buy cold-pressed 'extra virgin' olive oil, which is unrefined, dark green in colour and full of health-giving properties.

The polyunsaturated fats, found in seeds and nuts, and their oils as well as oily fish, are the most important fats to include in your child's diet, as they hold the key to immune function and proper brain development. Two of these polyunsaturated fats are essential. They are called alpha-linolenic acid and linoleic acid (otherwise known as omega 3 and omega 6 fats). The Family Tree of Fats (opposite) shows their different sources.

Starting your child on a daily intake of flaxseed oil at an early age is a good way to ensure adequate intake of the most important one, alpha-linolenic acid. I call it the most important because it is the most commonly deficient of the two. Flaxseed oil is made from linseeds (called flaxseeds in the United States) and can be given to your child from six months old. The dosage I recommend is 1 teaspoon a day from six months to two years, 2 teaspoons for two- to three-year-olds and 1 tablespoon for three plus. You should buy cold-pressed flaxseed oil from a healthfood shop. It comes in a dark bottle or container and you should keep it refrigerated to stop it going rancid. One particularly good brand is Omega Nutrition Flaxseed Oil (see Resources for suppliers). You can either add it to food before serving or slip it into a warm (not hot) drink at night. If your child dislikes the taste, you may have to be sneaky. My latest trick is to warm some rice milk and then place the milk, a banana and the oil in a food processor. This makes a delicious milkshake, boosts their fruit intake and blends the oil so that it goes largely undetected!

# THE FAMILY TREE OF FATS

**Saturated**
Butter, hard
cheese, palm
and coconut oil,
fatty meat

**Unsaturated**

**Trans fats**
Hydrogenated oils
such as margarines
and industrially
hardened fats. These
are found in biscuits,
pies, pastries, cakes
and crisps

**Monounsaturated**
Olive oil, rapeseed
oil, avocados, nuts
and seeds

**Polyunsaturated**
Vegetable oils, nuts,
seeds and oily fish

**Omega 6**
(derived from linoleic acid)
Sunflower, safflower, corn,
soya, evening primrose oils
and sesame seeds. Also
found in smaller amounts
in peanuts and peanut oil
and olive oil

**Omega 3**
(derived from
alpha-linolenic acid)
Flaxseed oil, green
leafy vegetables,
pumpkin seeds,
walnuts and walnut
oil. Also found in
oily fish: salmon,
herring, sardine,
mackerel, pilchard
and fresh tuna. In
smaller amounts it
is found in soya oil
and rapeseed oil

Finally, some especially bad fats worth mentioning are trans fats. Hydrogenated margarines are the worst source of these trans fats. Through a chemical process using extremely high temperatures, hydrogenation turns liquid vegetable oils into solid margarines. This process damages the oils and destroys their nutritional value. Processed foods also contain these harmful fats, the worst culprits being crisps, pastries, pies and some biscuits. You can now buy unhydrogenated vegetable margarines, which are healthy alternatives and these are good for spreading and for those on a dairy-free diet (see Resources).

## SUMMARY

1. Only serve lean red meat (beef or lamb) once a week to reduce saturated fat intake. Offer poultry, game and fish as healthier options. Avoid cured pork entirely (ham, bacon, salami), as it is too high in salt and nitrates.

2. Include oily fish in your child's diet at least once a week for beneficial polyunsaturated fats.

3. Introduce flaxseed oil supplementation from the age of six months.

4. Only fry with olive oil or a little butter which are heat-stable.

5. Avoid processed foods, biscuits, pastries, cakes and crisps which contain hydrogenated or 'trans fats'.

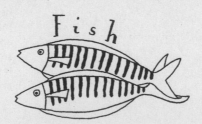

# Carbohydrate

Carbohydrate is the body's major source of fuel. There are two main forms: refined carbohydrates, like sugar, honey, malt, sweets and most refined foods; and complex carbohydrates, as in whole grains, vegetables and fresh fruit. Refined carbohydrates tend to produce a sudden burst of energy, followed by a slump (due to the fact that they cause a sudden rise, then fall, in blood sugar level). This can cause mood swings, irritability, temper tantrums and, inevitably, tears – the symptoms that most parents dread at the end of a birthday party! Complex carbohydrates provide more sustained, slow-release energy and are therefore much better all round. Refined foods describes most white foods: white bread, white flour, white rice, white pasta, white sugar, and anything made with white flour, like biscuits, cakes, crackers, etc. All these foods have been stripped of the fibre and the germ of the grain. In doing so, they have also removed as much as 80 per cent of the minerals in the whole grain.

## Percentage of minerals lost in refining flour

| | | | |
|---|---|---|---|
| Calcium | 60% | Iron | 75.6% |
| Phosphorus | 70.9% | Cobalt | 88.5% |
| Magnesium | 84.7% | Copper | 67.9% |
| Potassium | 77% | Zinc | 77.7% |
| Sodium | 78.3% | Selenium | 15.9% |
| Chromium | 98% | Molybdenum | 48% |
| Manganese | 85.8% | | |

## Healthy and unhealthy carbohydrates

| *Unhealthy carbohydrates* | *Healthy carbohydrates* |
| --- | --- |
| White sugar and anything made with it: | Fruit |
| | Vegetables |
| Sweets | Fresh juices (fruit and vegetable) |
| Biscuits | Home-made biscuits and cakes |
| Cakes | (made with fruit and fruit sugars) |
| Jellies | Naturally sweetened puddings |
| Soft drinks | |
| Jams | |
| White flour and anything made from it: | Wholemeal flour |
| | Wholemeal pasta |
| Bread | Wholemeal bread |
| Pasta | Brown rice |
| Crackers | Whole-grain rye crackers |
| Pastry | Jacket potatoes |
| White rice | Wholemeal pie cases |
| Processed breakfast cereals | Whole-grain breakfast cereals |
| | Porridge oats |
| | Pulses |

### SUMMARY

1. Offer 4–9 daily servings of healthy carbohydrates to your child.
2. Look in your cupboards, and if it's white – throw it out!

# Fibre

Fibre is an essential part of your child's diet. Not only does it slow down the release of sugars into the bloodstream, but it also helps to maintain the health of the digestive tract by creating bulk and thereby preventing constipation. There are two types of fibre: soluble and insoluble. Soluble fibre can be found in fruits and vegetables, and grains such as oats. It is the best type of fibre for your child. The most common type of insoluble fibre is wheat and wheat bran. However, insoluble fibre can be extremely abrasive on the digestive tract. Giving high-fibre cereals (like All Bran) or adding wheat bran to food is therefore not recommended for babies or young children.

By making sure that your child has enough soluble fibre in his diet, you will be helping to prevent many Western diseases such as heart disease, bowel cancer and diabetes as well as digestive disorders such as constipation, haemorrhoids, diverticulitis and irritable bowel syndrome. All these diseases have been linked with a low-fibre diet. Good sources of fibre are apples, pears, carrots, dried fruit, sweet potatoes, pulses, wholemeal bread, oats and brown rice.

## SUMMARY

1. Use whole grains instead of refined grains wherever possible as a good source of fibre and minerals, e.g. wholemeal bread instead of white bread, porridge oats rather than Ready Brek, and brown rice instead of white rice.

2. Once your child has teeth, offer hard fruits like apples and pears with the skins on. (Peel if not organic, to remove pesticide residues.)

3. Offer fruit and raw vegetables as high-fibre snacks.

## Water

Around 70 per cent of our body is composed of it and we can live for only two or three days without it. Water should therefore constitute the single most important element of your child's diet. Without sufficient water, they will become dehydrated and tired, and their digestive systems will be clogged and inefficient.

Offering water from an early age is the way to get your child interested in it. Water for a baby should be clean and pure, so tap water should ideally be filtered before being boiled. This will remove the majority of pollutants and chemicals that may be in your drinking water. Please do not fall into the trap of using baby juices which are often nothing more than coloured and sugared water with a little vitamin C thrown in for good measure. For the first two years of life your child only needs to drink either an appropriate milk or water. After this time, introducing very diluted 100 per cent fruit juices or concentrates is fine, though you may find that your child actually prefers to stick with water. Keep away from the squashes and fruit juice drinks even if the labels declare 'high' juice content, as they contain colours, sugar and artificial sweeteners which are not suitable for young children.

Fruit and vegetables are about 90 per cent water and provide water in a form that is very easy for the body to use, whilst at the same time providing the body with a high percentage of its vitamins and minerals. Make sure that your child eats five or more servings of fruit and vegetables a day.

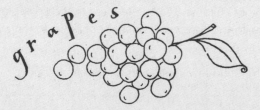

**SUMMARY**

**1.** Filter your tap water for all your family's drinking water.

**2.** Avoid baby juice drinks and fruit squashes, and stick to filtered water.

**3.** Encourage your child to have at least five servings of fruit and vegetables a day.

# Vitamins and minerals

Vitamins are needed in much smaller amounts than fat, protein or carbohydrate but are just as essential for health. Without vitamins, we can develop deficiency diseases such as scurvy, beri beri and rickets. Vitamins create energy, boost the immune system, maintain the brain and the nervous system, make healthy skin and hair, protect arteries and balance hormones.

Vitamins are separated into two groups: the water-soluble (B and C complex), and the fat-soluble (A, D, E and K). Water-soluble vitamins cannot be stored by the body so foods containing these should be eaten daily. They can also be easily destroyed by boiling, so try to preserve them by offering raw vegetables or lightly steaming them instead of boiling them. Another good way to preserve the vitamin content is to stir-fry vegetables quickly, as in Chinese Stir-fry with Tofu (page 150).

Minerals are also required for body processes to happen and they are divided into two groups: the macro-minerals, like calcium, magnesium, phosphorus and iron, which are needed in larger quantities; and the trace elements, like zinc, chromium, selenium and manganese, which we need only in tiny amounts. The Appendix gives details of the role performed by each vitamin or mineral, the symptoms of deficiency and the amount required to prevent deficiency.

## WHERE DO I FIND WHAT?

| Vitamins (technical names) | Good sources |
| --- | --- |
| Vitamin A (from retinol in animal foods or beta-carotene in plant foods) | Retinol: liver, oily fish, egg yolk, butter and cheese Beta-carotene: carrots, squashes, apricots, melon, and green leafy vegetables |
| Vitamin C (ascorbic acid) | Fruits and vegetables, especially citrus fruits, strawberries, kiwi fruit, blackcurrants and potatoes |
| Vitamin B1 (thiamin) | Liver, wheatgerm, whole grains, fortified breakfast cereals, potatoes, nuts and pulses |
| Vitamin B2 (riboflavin) | Yogurt, eggs, poultry, game, fish, wheatgerm |
| Vitamin B3 (niacin) | Poultry, lean meat, pulses, potatoes, whole grains, nuts, yeast extract |
| Vitamin B5 (pantothenic acid) | Contained in all meat and vegetable foods, particularly liver, dried fruits and nuts |

| Vitamins (technical names) | Good sources |
| --- | --- |
| Vitamin B6 (pyridoxine) | Poultry, game, fish, eggs, whole grains, nuts, bananas, yeast extract and soya beans |
| Vitamin B12 (cyanocobalamin) | Foods of animal origin, such as poultry, fish, eggs and dairy products, as well as fortified foods like cereals and vegetable margarines |
| Biotin | Liver, peanut butter, egg yolk, yeast extract, green leafy vegetables |
| Folic Acid (folate) | All green leafy vegetables like broccoli, Brussel sprouts, kale, cabbage, spinach, watercress and pak choi, as well as liver, wheatgerm and pulses |
| Vitamin D (calciferols) | Oily fish, like salmon, sardines and fresh tuna, and eggs and fortified margarines |
| Vitamin E (tocopherols) | Vegetable oils, wheatgerm, nuts, seeds, avocado |
| Vitamin K | Green leafy vegetables, especially green cabbage, broccoli and Brussel sprouts |

## Minerals

|  | *Good sources* |
|---|---|
| *Calcium* | Milk and dairy products, fortified soya products, tinned sardines, green leafy vegetables, molasses and sesame seeds |
| *Magnesium* | Whole-grain cereals, wheatgerm, pulses, nuts, seeds, dried fruits and green vegetables |
| *Potassium* | Avocados, fresh and dried fruit, seeds and nuts, bananas, citrus fruit, potatoes and pulses |
| *Chromium* | Liver, egg yolk, seafood, whole-grain cereals, molasses and cheese |
| *Iron* | Liver, poultry, game, lean meat, sardines, egg yolk, dark green leafy vegetables, molasses |
| *Zinc* | Seafood, poultry, game, lean red meat, sunflower seeds, peanuts, whole grains |
| *Selenium* | Seafood, Brazil nuts, avocados, seeds |
| *Manganese* | Whole grains, nuts, brown rice and pulses |

# HEALTH-MAKERS AND HEALTH-BREAKERS
## Health-makers

- Fresh fruits (preferably organic), especially eaten raw

- Fresh vegetables (preferably organic) and sprouted seeds and beans, especially eaten raw

- 100 per cent whole-grain bread and pastas, whole-grain cereals such as porridge made from oats, muesli and granola (but read the labels and watch out for hidden sugars)

- Fresh organic fruit and vegetable juices (diluted with water)

- Pulses, such as red lentils, and chickpeas (e.g. hummus)

- Organic cheeses in moderate quantities (provided no milk allergies present)

- Dried fruits (naturally dried, not sulphur-dried), such as raisins, dates, sultanas and apricots which are all rich in iron

- Nuts (make sure they are ground to a powder for young children) and seeds

- Organic eggs

- Poultry and game

- Fish (especially oily ones like mackerel, herring, fresh salmon, sardine and tuna – the canning process damages the essential fats)

- Unhydrogenated margarines like Vitaquell or Vitaseig (see Resources) or a little butter for spreading

- Extra-virgin olive oil for cooking and dressings

- Flaxseed oil, added to food in dressings or shakes

## Health-breakers

- White bread, rolls, pastries and pies
- White pasta (spaghetti, macaroni, etc)
- Cakes and biscuits made from white flour
- Jelly (except home-made fruit jelly)
- Jams (except 100 per cent fruit jams)
- Tinned fruit in syrup
- Packet and tinned soups
- Chips (except home-made)
- Crisps
- Fizzy drinks which contain sugar or artificial sweeteners
- Chocolate and sweets
- Artificial fruit drinks and squashes
- Cream and ice cream (except home made yogurt ice cream)
- Margarine and processed oils, golden in colour, found in supermarkets
- Caffeine, found in coffee, tea, chocolate, chocolate drinks and some fizzy drinks
- Salt (do not add salt to your cooking at all for this age group)

## How do I make sure my child is getting enough nutrients?

Although it is extremely useful to be aware of which foods contain the essential nutrients that your child needs, it would be almost impossible to analyse what your child was receiving in terms of vitamins and minerals every day. The easiest way to ensure that they get the maximum range of nutrients is to supply them with as varied a diet as you can. Follow the simple advice in this chapter and you will be supplying them with a nutrient-rich diet which is as close as possible to the government guidelines for recommended nutrient intakes.

I say 'as close as possible' because sadly our food does not contain the level of nutrients that it used to. With nutrient depletion in the soil due to intensive farming, and long-distance shipping and storage of fruits and vegetables, levels of nutrients have been steadily declining over the last 50 years. For this reason, I always recommend that every child over the age of six months receive a mutivitamin and mineral. This will ensure good levels of the essential nutrients required for optimal growth and development. By using a formula designed for babies and very young children you will never run the risk of giving your child too much.

For babies from six months to two years there are specially designed liquid and powdered multiformulations (see Resources). From two to five years old, I recommend a good chewable multivitamin and mineral (see Resources). These are formulated so that you give one chewable for every two years of age. Therefore a four-year-old would be having two chewables a day. Always give supplements at mealtimes when they will be better assimilated with the food.

Variety is definitely the key to a healthy diet. Many of us tend to rely on a few foods which we eat repeatedly on a daily basis. A typical young child's diet will consist of a wheat-based cereal for breakfast (like Weetabix) and some toast. For lunch he might have pasta with a tomato and cheese sauce, followed by a yogurt; and then for tea a ham sandwich, maybe with some fruit and a biscuit. This type of repetitive diet is very common but is over-reliant on wheat and dairy products, and will restrict the nutrients your child is receiving.

A better variation on the above would be oat porridge, a banana and rye crackers for breakfast; corn pasta with a vegetable sauce, followed by a yogurt for lunch; and then a choice of sandwiches and fruit for tea. You have not changed the menu a great deal but you have included four different grains rather than one, increased the amount of fruit and vegetables in the diet, and included a variety of flavours and textures. In this way you are exposing your child to a much greater range of nutrients and also helping to prevent any food intolerances developing which can occur if too much of the same food is eaten too often.

## What is a serving?

When you first introduce solid food to your baby at around six months, he will only be having tiny tastes but will quickly progress onto bigger meals. As a guide, a baby of 6–9 months can eat 1–4 tablespoons at each meal and this will consist largely of fruit, vegetables and grains in purée form. Babies of 9–12 months will, on average, be eating 3–6 tablespoons of food at each meal, divided into a savoury purée, followed by a fruit pudding. Remember that this is only to give you a very rough idea of quantities. Every baby's appetite is different – let them be your guide.

Once your baby reaches the ripe old age of one, it is easier to quantify his diet using the healthy eating pyramid above. A serving for a 1–5-year-old represents any helping which is more than a couple of mouthfuls. Some toddlers will eat a whole piece of toast at a meal, while others prefer only a couple of soldier slices. A serving of fruit for a one-year-old can, for example, be an apple quarter. By the time they reach four, they will probably

# THE HEALTHY EATING PYRAMID FOR CHILDREN

Here is an at-a-glance view of how to achieve the right balance in your child's diet.

**Fats and oils**
Butter, olive oil, seed and nut oils, unhydrogenated margarines

— Use sparingly

**Good-quality protein foods**
Poultry, meat, fish, liver, nuts, seeds, cheese, yogurt, lentils, quinoa, tofu (soya)

— 3–5 servings a day

5+ servings a day —

**Fruit and vegetables**
Dark green leafy vegetables like broccoli, kale, cabbage, watercress, Brussel sprouts, spinach and green beans; root vegetables like carrot, sweet potato, parsnip, turnip, potato, beetroot, swede; salad vegetables like tomatoes, peppers, spring onions, celery, cucumber, lettuce, sprouted beans and seeds, etc; fruit, such as apples, pears, bananas, melon, berries and citrus fruit and their juices

4–9 servings a day

**Carbohydrates and fibre**
Whole-grain breads and pastas, brown rice, oats, barley, rye, corn, millet, buckwheat, pulses, potato

**Water/fluids**
600–1800 ml (1–3 pints) a day, depending on age and weather, offered throughout the day

be eating a whole apple. Again, there are no hard and fast rules. As long as your child is growing and thriving, he is eating enough. Children have a very strong natural survival instinct which makes them eat when they are hungry. If they are not hungry, they will not eat, despite any amount of coaxing and cajoling. Let them decide.

On the opposite page I have put together a sample day's menu for a one-year-old, using the healthy eating pyramid as a guide. As you can see, all the dietary targets are reached. This shows how easy it is to give your child enough of the right foods to keep him healthy.

# Preparing food for your family

## What equipment do I need?

Many of the recipes in this book can be adapted for bulk cooking, baby purées for the freezer, or feeding a whole family. Therefore I highly recommend a few essential pieces of equipment for the kitchen.

### A food processor

Look for a food processor which has a small bowl attachment inside. This allows you to purée small amounts of food at a time, which is useful if you have only one small mouth to feed. However, if you do not have one in the kitchen and want a cheaper option, there are now some very good hand-held blenders and moulis available.

### A steamer

I'm a great fan of steaming vegetables. Steaming preserves the vitamins and minerals in the vegetables better than any other

# Sample day's menu for a one-year-old

## MENU

### BREAKFAST
Oat Porridge (page 106) with banana and tahini (sesame seed spread)
Wholemeal toast fingers with 100 per cent fruit jam
Appropriate milk to drink

### SNACK
Apple or pear slices

### LUNCH
Fish Pie (page 170), broccoli and carrots
Fruit Smoothie (page 185)
Water to drink

### SNACK
Magical Muffin (page 201)

### TEA
Corn Spaghetti with Quick and Easy Pasta Sauce (page 136)
Finger salad
Soya yogurt
Water to drink

### BEDTIME
Appropriate milk to drink and a rice cake

### TOTAL SERVINGS
Protein = 5 servings
Fruit and veg = 6 servings
Carbohydrate = 6 servings

cooking method. When you are preparing fruit and vegetable purées for your 6–12-month-old baby you will initially need to cook the vegetables until they are very soft; but, for toddlers and the adults in the family, veggies al dente will look nicer, taste nicer and be much healthier all round. A cheaper alternative to a steamer is using a colander over a pan of boiling water with a tight-fitting lid to prevent too much steam escaping.

### Measuring spoons and measuring cups

Because most mothers are too busy to keep weighing ingredients when cooking, I often use measuring cups and measuring spoons in the recipes. They are so much quicker and easier to use; they are also very cheap and are available at good supermarkets.

### Ice cube trays and freezer bags

These are an essential part of the equipment needed for preparing your baby's first meals. They are used for freezing fruit and vegetables purées, as explained below, and will make your life so much easier in terms of meal planning.

## Freezing baby foods

The best type of ice cube trays to buy are the ones that you can twist once frozen. These allow the easiest extraction and also tend to hold more purée. Pour boiling water over the ice cube trays to sterilise them before using. Cook and purée the fruit or vegetables (as described in the recipes on pages 86–94), scoop the purées into the trays, cover and allow to cool. Once cooled, place in the freezer until set hard. When they are frozen, twist the cubes out of the trays and place them in freezer bags labelled with the date on which they were made, so that you do not give your baby frozen food over the expiry limits suggested opposite. All recipes indicate whether or not they can be frozen.

In order to serve your baby a meal from the freezer you will need to do the following. Remove the relevant number of ice cubes from the freezer and allow them to defrost at room temperature for several hours. A fruit or vegetable purée may only take an hour to defrost, whereas a mixed meal of meat or fish and vegetables will take considerably longer. Once defrosted, heat gently in a pan and cool before offering it to your baby. Do not refreeze foods that have already been frozen and do not reheat foods more than once.

## Freezing Times

**The temperature of your freezer should be a minimum of 0°F (−18°C).**

| | |
|---|---|
| Fruit purées | 6 months |
| Vegetable purées | 3 months |
| Meat, cooked | 3 months |
| Fish, cooked | 2 months |
| Pulses | 2 months |
| Grains | 2 months |

## Healthiest cooking methods

- Steaming
- Stir-frying
- Oven-baking
- Grilling

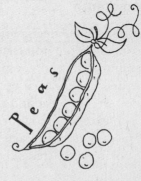

# Superfoods for the larder

Throughout this book, you will come across many new foods some of which you may not have heard of before. You will find a list of the most important ones and their health benefits below. But, before you rush out and restock your cupboards, remember that some of these foods do not have very long shelf lives. It's therefore best to do your buying in stages, restocking as and when you decide to make particular dishes. You will then be able to use the ingredient several times without wasting any. Some of these foods are available from supermarkets, some from healthfood shops and some from the suppliers listed under Resources (pages 230–232).

## Agar agar

A vegetarian alternative to gelatin, which is advisable in the light of the BSE scare. It is derived from sea algae and is available in powder, flake, strip and strand form. Dissolve 2 teaspoons powder or 1 tablespoon flakes in 600 ml (1 pint) boiling water or unsweetened fruit juice to make a firm jelly. Simmer the solution for 1–2 minutes whilst whisking vigorously to dissolve the agar agar thoroughly. **Suitable from one year.**

## Amaranth

An ancient Aztec grain, which is now making a comeback. It contains more iron than any other plant and all eight essential amino acids and is especially high in lysine. When combined with other grains, it becomes a high-quality protein food, superior even to meat and other animal products. For this reason it is an excellent food for growing children and nursing mothers. The only disadvantage is that it is still quite expensive. See the Cooking with Grains chart (page 42). **Suitable from six months.**

## Apricots

Dried, unsulphured apricots are a very good source of iron. For this reason they make a good weaning food, combined with cereals or other fruits. They are also an excellent natural sweetener for puddings and fruit spreads but remember to use them sparingly to protect your children's teeth. Apricots which are treated with sulphur dioxide (E220) to preserve their rich orange colour may cause allergic reactions in some individuals. They are a suspected trigger in asthma attacks and should therefore be avoided. **Suitable from six months.**

## Arrowroot

Can be used as a thickener in place of cornflour. It is made from the cassava plant. **Suitable from six months.**

## Baking powder

Raising agent used in baking cakes, breads and biscuits. Make sure you buy an aluminium-free brand. Aluminium-containing brands will include sodium aluminium sulfate in their list of ingredients. **Suitable from one year.**

## Barley

A gluten grain that makes an excellent addition to soups and stews. Pot barley available in healthfood shops is of a superior quality to the polished pearl barley which you find on supermarket shelves. It is believed to have anti-viral properties and has traditionally been used as barley water to treat digestive and urinary complaints in some parts of the world. To make barley water, wash 1 tablespoon pot barley and simmer gently for half an hour in 600 ml (1 pint) water. Strain the water, cool and sip slowly.

To make barley for a meal, see the Cooking with Grains chart (page 42). **Suitable from nine months**.

## Barley malt syrup

A mild, natural alternative to sugar. Barley malt syrup is made from barley sprouts and water which are cooked to a syrup. It is only 40 per cent as sweet as sugar and can be used in place of sugar in baking. **Suitable from nine months**.

## Brewer's yeast

An excellent source of B vitamins, protein, and valuable minerals like iron, zinc and potassium. A useful addition to an energy shake or when sprinkled on stews and soups prior to serving. Brewer's yeast is high in purines which may tax the kidneys of young babies and is therefore **unsuitable for those under 12 months**.

## Buckwheat

The staple food of Russia and Poland. Although treated as a grain, it is in fact a nut, produced by the flowering thistle plant. Buckwheat comes in groats, which can be bought ready-roasted and used in soups, stews and pilafs. Buckwheat flour is an excellent alternative to wheat flour and makes delicious pancakes.

To cook buckwheat as a grain, see the Cooking with Grains chart (page 42). **Suitable from six months**.

## Carob flour

A superb alternative to chocolate. Carob powder is made from the seeds of the Mediterranean carob tree and is naturally sweet. It is free from caffeine, rich in B vitamins and some minerals and is similar in taste to cocoa. It can be used in chocolate-type drinks, puddings and treats. If substituting for cocoa powder in a recipe, use half the suggested quantity of cocoa. **Suitable from one year.**

## Dates

Dates provide another excellent substitute for sugar and are rich in iron. The best way of using dates is to buy them pitted (without stones) and make a purée (page 90). This can be stored in an airtight jar for a couple of weeks in the fridge and used in biscuits or cakes or spread thinly on rice cakes or in sandwiches. **Suitable from six months.**

## Flaxseed oil

The easiest vegetable source of omega 3 essential fatty acids to use in a young child's diet, especially when added to drinks and shakes. **Suitable from six months.**

## Flours

**Wholewheat flour:** Useful in baking, binding and dusting. (**One year**)

**Unbleached, white, plain flour:** Useful for making sauces. This flour contains 72 per cent of the whole grain and fewer additives than the bleached version. (**One year**)

**Rice flour:** Useful for gluten-free baking. (**Six months**)

**Potato flour:** Good wheat flour substitute in casseroles and soups. (**Nine months**)

**Soya flour:** High-protein flour which has a strong taste. Useful to boost the protein and nutrient content of a recipe. Not suitable for making sauces. (**Nine months**)

**Buckwheat flour:** Gluten-free flour useful in making pancakes and for dusting foods in place of wheat flour. (**Six months**)

**Gram flour:** Chickpea flour with a high protein content. (**Six months**)

**'All purpose flour':** Created by Terence Stamp and Elizabeth Buxton as a wheat-free alternative. Containing barley, rice, millet and maize, it is a very good but expensive alternative to wheat flour. (**Nine months**)

## Fruit juice concentrates

Useful sugar substitutes for the storecupboard. Can be diluted 1:10 with water as a fruit juice drink, frozen into lollies or used in baking as an alternative to sugar. The most common ones are apple juice concentrate and apple and blackcurrant juice concentrate. Apple and blackcurrant is excellent in terms of vitamin C content. **Suitable from one year.**

## Fruit spreads

100 per cent fruit spreads are a good substitute for sugary jams. They come in all sorts of wonderful flavours, such as peach and passionfruit, blackcurrant, raspberry, apricot and pear, and are available in some supermarkets as well as healthfood stores. Use sparingly on toast or as a sweetener for a pudding. **Suitable from six months.**

## Garlic

Garlic is anti-bacterial, anti-fungal and anti-viral. It is best to add some garlic at the end as cooking reduces its antibiotic effect. **Suitable from six months.**

## Lecithin

A soya-derived fat emulsifier which adds to the smoothness and creaminess of some recipes. A rich source of phosphatidyl choline, an essential brain food. **Suitable from nine months**.

## Manuka honey (tea tree honey)

A must for all storecupboards, as it contains anti-bacterial and anti-viral properties. To soothe sore throats, put a teaspoon of honey into a cup, squeeze in the juice of half a lemon and fill with hot (not boiling) water. Allow to cool slightly and drink. Do not give honey to babies under one, as there is a risk of infection. **Suitable from one year**.

## Maple syrup (organic)

Another useful sugar substitute, in small quantities. **Suitable from one year**.

## Margarine

Unhydrogenated margarines available from healthfood stores are good substitutes for butter. There are now a number available that are designed for spreading and some that are stable enough to cook with. Most are now fortified with vitamins A, D and B12 and are therefore suitable for vegans. **Suitable from nine months**.

## Millet

A gluten-free grain which is alkaline in nature. It contains all eight essential amino acids and is a particularly good source of silicon, a mineral required for healthy bones, teeth, nails and hair. It comes as a grain or as flakes. Useful to have both. See the Cooking with Grains chart (page 42). **Suitable from six months**.

## Molasses

A by-product of sugar refining, molasses is renowned for its high mineral content. Weight for weight, crude blackstrap molasses contains more calcium than milk and more iron than eggs, as well as a high level of potassium. It is naturally sweet but has a distinctive, strong taste and so is only used in very small amounts. It can be used as a sugar substitute in baking, stews and cereals. **Suitable from six months**.

## Nuts

An excellent form of protein, fat, calcium and iron for vegetarians and vegans. Chopped mixed nuts are good for nut roasts, ground nuts are a useful addition to vegetable purées, and nut butters are delicious and wholesome on bread and rice crackers. Combining nuts with breads, grains and pulses will ensure that you receive all eight of the essential amino acids. My favourites for children are almonds and cashews and their butters. Peanut butter is fine in small amounts as long as there is no history of peanut allergy in your family. It is best to buy ground roasted peanuts with nothing else added, available at healthfood shops. Alternatively you can make your own (see page 181).

Never give whole nuts to children under five, as they can choke on them. Buy nuts in small quantities and use them quickly to prevent them becoming rancid. Keep them in a cool, dark place, ideally a lidded glass jar in the fridge. Never eat rancid nuts, as they can contain high levels of aflatotoxin, a mould, that can cause cancer. **Suitable from nine months**.

## Oats

A highly nutritious grain supplying plenty of calcium, magnesium, potassium and B vitamins. Oats do not contain gluten but they do contain a similar protein and therefore should not be given to babies where there is a history of coeliac disease. **Suitable from nine months.**

## Oils

These should be unrefined and cold-pressed to ensure a high-quality oil. Extra-virgin olive oil is my favourite for the store-cupboard. It is a monounsaturated oil which remains stable at high temperatures and is therefore a good oil to choose for sautéeing or stir-frying as well as using in dressings. Extra-virgin olive oil is dark green and comes from the first pressing of the olives with no additives. You can use cold-pressed, unrefined sunflower, safflower and walnut oil for baking and dressings but do not use these polyunsaturates for high-temperature cooking. At high temperatures these oils do not remain stable and will create free radicals which can damage your child's health. **Suitable from six months.**

## Parsley

A mega-superfood for the larder. It is a good source of vitamins A and C as well as calcium, iron and folic acid. Parsley flavours savoury dishes beautifully and is an excellent first fresh herb to introduce children to. Use plenty in your cooking, and always add some at the end to preserve its colour and nutrients. **Suitable from six months.**

## Pasta

There is now such a huge range of pastas available that you don't have to always serve wheat pasta at home. Why not try rice and vegetable pasta (**six months**), corn pasta (**nine months**), corn tagliatelle, spinach and barley pasta (**nine months**), garlic pasta, buckwheat pasta (**six months**) and chickpea pasta (**six months**), for example? They all tend to need less cooking time than wholewheat pasta and all have their own special flavours. You will find them in your local healthfood store, although some supermarkets are now stocking a wider variety.

### Popping corn

An excellent snack food for children. Make your own at home using a little olive oil in the bottom of the pan and adding a handful of corn. Cover the pan with a lid and wait till the corn starts popping. Keep shaking the pan until all the popping stops. The advantage of making it at home is that you can serve it with no sugar or salt added and children still love it. **Suitable from nine months.**

### Pulses

Buy pulses either dried (the cheapest way) or canned without sugar or salt. See Cooking with Pulses (page 41) for soaking and cooking times. My favourites are: green lentils, adzuki beans, red lentils, butter beans, flageolet beans, haricot beans and kidney beans. **Suitable from six months.**

### Quinoa

A South American grain which is rich in calcium and iron and an excellent meat and dairy alternative for vegans as it contains all eight of the essential amino acids. It must, however, be thoroughly washed before cooking to remove the bitter coating which can be harmful if eaten in large quantities. Quinoa can be used as an alternative to rice or millet – see the Cooking with Grains chart (page 42). **Suitable from six months.**

### Raisins

These are dried grapes and make excellent sweeteners for cereal dishes. Use only sun-dried versions without added chemicals. A box of raisins is a useful snack for children, but remember that they are still a highly concentrated food that can cause tooth decay if eaten on their own too frequently. **Suitable from six months**.

## Rice

A gluten-free grain which comes in many different guises. Always use brown rice which is unrefined and contains more nutrients – see the Cooking with Grains chart (page 42). It is available as long-grain, short-grain, sweet brown rice, rice flakes and rice flour. It is an excellent first food for babies in the form of Rice Porridge (page 95), and by using sweet brown rice you get a delicious Brown Rice Pudding (page 190). **Suitable from six months**.

## Rice milk

Rice water has traditionally been used as a remedy for infant diarrhoea in many countries. Rice milk, which is made from rice, filtered water, safflower oil and sea salt, is a delicious drink and dairy alternative. It is especially useful as a dairy alternative when your children have colds and infections as, unlike milk and dairy products, it will not increase their mucus congestion. However, it does not contain the same levels of calcium, fat or protein that dairy foods provide and these should therefore be supplied elsewhere in the diet (page 4). **Suitable from six months**.

## Seeds

Seeds have excellent nutrient contents and can be used in cereals, salads, soups, dips, spreads, grain dishes, toppings and burgers. Here are my favourite four for the larder. Keep them in the fridge and use them quickly to prevent the oils turning rancid.

**Sesame seeds:** Rich in vitamin B3, protein, iron, zinc, polyunsaturated fats and vitamin E. They also come as a paste called tahini which is a lovely nutty addition to soups and porridges and is also an ingredient in hummus. (**Nine months**)

**Sunflower seeds:** An excellent snack alternative, these seeds are packed full of protein, B vitamins and polyunsaturated fats. (**Nine months**)

**Pumpkin seeds:** Contain the highest level of zinc amongst the seeds as well as notable amounts of iron and calcium. (**Nine months**)

**Flaxseeds/linseeds:** Excellent source of omega 3 essential fatty acids. The best way to use them for children is to grind them up in a coffee grinder and sprinkle them on cereals. Also available as a concentrated oil which is extremely beneficial for skin complaints and constipation. (**Six months**)

## Semolina

Made from durum wheat, which is most commonly used to make pasta and gnocchi, semolina is soft wheat with the outer layer of the wheat berry removed. It is available in wholewheat or white versions and makes excellent puddings. **Suitable from one year.**

## Soya milk

A dairy alternative which comes in fortified, plain or organic versions. Buy an organic brand to ensure that it's not made from genetically modified soya beans. Fortified versions are essential for vegans and children who do not eat dairy products. **Suitable from nine months.**

## Sprouts

The cheapest powerhouses of nutrition. Sprouted seeds and beans are a terrific source of vitamins and minerals. Once sprouted, their nutritional value escalates. Oats contain 1300 per cent more vitamin B2 once sprouted, vitamin B6 goes up by 500 per cent, and folic acid by 600 per cent. A tablespoon of soya bean sprouts contains half the recommended adult requirement of vitamin C. Sprouting is cheap and easy, and your children will love helping you (see pages 38–40). Using organic seeds and pulses will get you the best results. **Suitable from nine months**.

## Tahini

Ground sesame seeds (see Seeds, above). **Suitable from nine months**.

## Tamari

A wheat-free soy sauce, lower in sodium than soy sauce. Bragg's Liquid Aminos (a brand of soy sauce) is also made from the tamari family. It is, however, unfermented, lower in sodium and contains all eight essential amino acids. Use sparingly in stir-fries. Do not give to a child under one as the sodium content is too high. **Suitable from one year**.

## Tofu

Tofu is soya bean curd made from soya milk. It is an excellent meat and dairy substitute, high in protein and low in fat. There are two types: silken and firm. Silken is more suitable for shakes and drinks; firm tofu can be drained, chopped and used as a meat alternative in stir-fries, risottos and stews. **Suitable from nine months**.

## Vegetable bouillon powder

A gluten-free, yeast-free vegetable stock powder. You can now get a low-salt version. It is the healthiest stock to use in your kitchen – free from additives and monosodium glutamate. As it comes in a powder form, you can use very little when cooking for children. Once you have tried it, you will never return to stock cubes (see Resources). **Suitable from nine months**.

## Wheatgerm

The germ of the wheat is what is left after it has been refined. So, rather like molasses, it is the best bit nutritionally. Wheatgerm is an excellent source of B vitamins, iron and vitamin E. Buy it raw and sprinkle on fruit salads or live yogurt or use it in cereal mixes. Keep it in the fridge as it can go rancid quickly. **Suitable from one year**.

# Seeds, pulses and grains

## Sprouting seeds

Sprouting is cheap and fun, and provides a vitamin-packed food to introduce your child to. When mine were very young I used to buy packs of organic sprouted seeds and pulses which they loved, but I soon realised it was a rather expensive way of doing it. Now we do it at home and the boys enjoy helping.

## What you will need

- Dried mung beans
- Colander
- A glass or china bowl

- A jam jar or seed tray

- Filtered or bottled water

- A tea towel, muslin or cheesecloth

- A sieve

## TEN STEPS TO PERFECT SPROUTS

**1.** Put 2 tablespoons dried mung beans into a bowl.

**2.** Remove any bits of stone or broken beans which will not sprout.

**3.** Fill the bowl with water and soak overnight (12–15 hours).

**4.** In the morning pour the beans into a sieve, rinse well and allow to drain over a colander for a few minutes.

**5.** Give them a gentle shake to get rid of any excess drips and transfer the seeds to the jam jar, cover with a tea towel, and put in a warm, dark place (like an airing cupboard or next to the boiler). They will take longer to sprout if it is not warm.

**6.** Twice a day, fill the jar with water and pour the seeds into the sieve to drain the water away. (If they sit in too much water they will rot rather than sprout.)

**7.** If it is very hot, you may have to rinse them in the middle of the day as well.

**8.** As the beans start sprouting, you will see little shoots appearing. Between the third and fifth day of sprouting (depending how long you want the sprouts to grow), pop them on a windowsill for a couple of hours for a dose of sunlight.

**9.** Rinse well and eat them straight away.

**10.** Your sprouts will be ready to eat within 3–5 days. They make a lovely addition to salads or you can add them to a stir-fry. Sprouts will keep for a few days in the fridge if you put them in a resealable plastic bag or airtight container.

## Sprouting chart

|  | Soaking time | Quantity of beans | Sprouting time |
| --- | --- | --- | --- |
| Alfalfa seeds | 6–8 hours | 2 tablespoons | 5–6 days |
| Mung beans | 12–15 hours | A handful | 3–5 days |
| Chickpeas | 15–18 hours | 2 handfuls | 3–4 days |
| Lentils | 12–15 hours | A handful | 3–5 days |
| Adzuki beans | 12–15 hours | 2 handfuls | 3–5 days |

Once you have mastered these, you can move onto sprouting sesame, sunflower and pumpkin seeds and other beans.

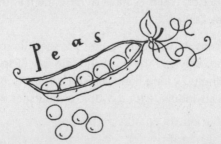

# Cooking with pulses

If you buy dried pulses, which is certainly the cheapest way, you will need to rinse and sometimes soak them before cooking. All pulses need twice their own volume of water to cook in. The first ten minutes' cooking of all the pulses, except the lentils and split peas, should be done at a fast boil. This destroys any enzymes that can cause tummy upsets.

## Soaking, preparing and cooking pulses

| Pulse | Soaking time | Preparation | Cooking time (average) |
|---|---|---|---|
| Green lentils | None | Rinse well | 40 minutes |
| Red lentils | None | Rinse well | 20 minutes |
| Split peas | None | Rinse well | 40 minutes |
| Adzuki beans | Overnight | Rinse and drain | 45 minutes |
| Butter beans | Overnight | Rinse and drain | 90 minutes |
| Flageolet beans | Overnight | Rinse and drain | 45 minutes |
| Haricot beans | Overnight | Rinse and drain | 60 minutes |
| Red kidney beans | Overnight | Rinse and drain | 50 minutes |
| Soya beans | Overnight | Rinse and drain | 2–2½ hours |
| Chickpeas | Overnight | Rinse and drain | 90 minutes |

Cooked pulses can be kept in an airtight container in the fridge for several days or can be frozen. It is best to freeze them on trays and then pack them in small containers. This way, you can just add a couple of handfuls to a recipe without any preparation.

## Cooking with grains

Wash the grains well and add them to boiling water for the time specified below. The size of the cup does not matter. It can be a teacup, mug or American measuring cup – it's just an easy way to describe how much water you need to add when cooking the grains. For variety and a fuller flavour, it is sometimes nice to cook the grains in vegetable stock as in Herby Millet (page 141).

### Cooking grains

| Grain | Amount of grain | Amount of water | Cooking time |
| --- | --- | --- | --- |
| Amaranth | 1 cup | 2 cups | 10–15 minutes |
| Barley | 1 cup | 4 cups | 60–75 minutes |
| Brown rice | 1 cup | 2 cups | 25–40 minutes |
| Buckwheat | 1 cup | 2 cups | 15–20 minutes |
| Millet | 1 cup | 3 cups | 15–20 minutes |
| Quinoa | 1 cup | 2 cups | 10–15 minutes |

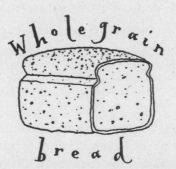

# Label watching

The first ingredient on the label is always the largest component, regardless of what the product is called. If water comes first, for example, there will be more water in that product than anything else. Once you know this, you realise that many commercially produced foods are poor value – both in terms of money and nutrition.

## Quick label reference guide

This chart, designed by the British Heart Foundation, is an excellent guide to reading labels.

| A lot | A little |
|---|---|
| 20 g fat | 3 g fat |
| 5 g saturates | 1 g saturates |
| 10 g sugars | 2 g sugars |
| 0.5 g sodium | 0.1 g sodium |

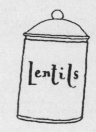

For foods your children eat in large amounts (e.g. breakfast cereals) you need to look at the amount per serving. For foods eaten in small amounts, look at the 100 g (4 oz) information on the pack.

## Look out for hidden sugar in labels

Sugar may be included in both sweet and savoury meals. It may be labelled as sucrose, glucose, maltose, dextrose, glucose syrup, lactose, corn syrup, hydrolysed starch, inverted sugar, fructose or concentrated fruit juice. Remember that 1 level teaspoon of sugar (5 ml) is equivalent to 4 g in weight. Look at a few labels when you are at the supermarket. Dividing the sugar weight by

4 will tell you how many teaspoons of sugar there are in 100 g (4 oz), or one serving. It can be quite a shock when you discover that, for example, there is as much as 4 teaspoons of sugar in some fromage frais and yogurts designed for children.

## E numbers

There are many books on this subject. Some E numbers, derived from vitamin sources, are good for us; and some are bad. Here is a list of the good E numbers which you may find easier to remember than the bad.

Colourings:   E101 (Riboflavin), E160 (Carotene)

Antioxidants: E300–E304 (Ascorbates)

              E306–E309 (Tocopherols)

Emulsifiers,
stabilisers,
and others:   E322 (Lecithin), E375 (Nicotinic acid), E440 (Pectin)

## Avoid fillers

Starch, modified starch, cornflour (maize flour), maltodextrin, rice flour, soya flour, gelatin, pectin and vegetable gums are all 'fillers'. These low-nutrient ingredients are there to replace 'real' food and serve to thicken and absorb water in order to increase the bulk of the food. One recent study on the effects of modified starch on infants showed raised frequency of loose stools. Modified starch is made from chemically treated cornflour.

## Avoid nitrates

These preservatives can be found in all cured foods and some smoked foods, especially sausages, ham and bacon. Nitrates convert to nitrosamines in the stomach, which are suspected of being carcinogenic (cancer-forming). If you want to include pork in your child's diet, find a good organic butcher who does not use nitrates in his meat (see Resources).

## Why say no to sugar?

Sugar has a powerful depressive effect on the immune system. Research has shown that as little as 6 teaspoons of sugar a day can reduce the effectiveness of the immune system by 25 per cent.

Considering that there are up to 4 teaspoons of sugar in an average fruit yogurt, 2½ teaspoons in half a tin of baked beans and as many as 8 teaspoons in a small bar of chocolate, you can see how much sugar can sneak into a child's daily diet. If your baby, toddler or young child seems to have endless colds, picking up one bug after another, you may find that cutting out sugar is all that is needed to give his immune system a boost.

### Hidden sugar in foods

| Food | Serving size | Quantity of sugar (in teaspoons) |
|------|------|------|
| Digestive biscuits | 2 biscuits | 1 |
| Fruit yogurt | 1 small pot | 4 |
| Baked beans | ½ medium can | 2½ |
| Tinned sweetcorn | ⅓ large tin | 2 |
| Tomato ketchup | 2 teaspoons | ½ |
| Milk chocolate | 1 small bar | 6½ |
| Smarties | 1 tube | 7½ |
| Ice cream | 1 scoop | 2 |

> **Sugar alternatives**
>
> Fruit juices and juice concentrates
> Dried fruit purées
> Fructose
> Molasses
> Barley malt syrup
> Maple syrup (in moderation)
> Date syrup
> Rice malt syrup

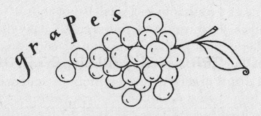

## Watch out for salt!

Did you know that a serving of Cornflakes or Rice Krispies contains more salt than a packet of ready-salted crisps?

New government guidelines reveal that young children should consume no more than 1.75 g (1750 mg) of salt a day. That is one-third of the adult recommendation of 6 g (6000 mg). Too much salt puts a strain on the kidneys, and can increase calcium excretion and thus add to the risk of developing osteoporosis in later life.

Most of the salt we consume is hidden and it is therefore important to know which foods contain it. Food labels list sodium in the ingredients. To calculate the salt (sodium chloride) content, multiply the sodium figure by 2.5.

## Hidden salt in foods

| Food | Salt content |
| --- | --- |
| Bread (all types) | 500 mg per slice |
| Cheddar cheese | 335 mg in 50 g (2 oz) |
| Cornflakes | 900 mg per bowl |
| Crisps | 675 mg per packet |
| Sausages | 1250 mg per 50 g (two small) |
| Fish fingers | 475 mg per 50 g (two small) |
| Digestive biscuits | 375 mg per 25 g (two biscuits) |

# Avoid genetically modified foods

There has been a great deal of publicity regarding the advent of genetically modified foods in our diet. In my opinion, quite apart from the environmental impact of these foods, there is not enough research to satisfy me that they are safe for children (or, indeed, adults) to consume. I therefore do not recommend that you allow your children to become part of a huge genetic experiment. What is more, exposing small children to GM soya may also increase the incidence of allergy to soya amongst children.

To avoid genetically modified foods, eat as much organic food as possible and stick to organic sources of the culprit foods wherever possible. Organic food is not currently allowed to contain GM ingredients. Avoid processed foods, which can contain many GM ingredients.

Baby Organix, Cow and Gate, Hipp, Milupa and Olvarit are five baby food manufacturers who do not knowingly use GM ingredients or processing aids.

## Hidden GM ingredients

The following foods may be derived from genetically modified soya beans and tomatoes:

| | |
|---|---|
| Lecithin | Soya flour |
| Vegetable oil | Soya milks |
| Vegetable fat | Soya products (tofu, tempeh, |
| Corn oil | textured vegetable protein) |
| Soya oil | Yeast products |
| Cornflour | Hydrogenated vegetable fat |
| Modified starch | Soya protein isolates |
| Modified cornflour | Tomato purée |
| HVP (hydrolised vegetable | Maltodextrin |
| protein) | |

# Food allergies and intolerance

There is a great deal of controversy over food allergies. Classic food allergies, which are called Type I allergies (IgE), involve an immediate response from the immune system and can be extremely dangerous, if not fatal. The foods that can cause this type of reaction are nuts, seeds, egg, fish and soya products.

The second type of food allergy is called a food intolerance or food sensitivity. It is called a Type II reaction (IgG) and does not necessarily involve any immune response at all. These types of food reactions can be difficult to isolate but being aware of the common symptoms is a good place to start. Food intolerances can build up over time and are usually caused by foods that are eaten recurrently. The most common culprits are wheat and dairy products, which are often eaten several times a day from a very early age.

Here are some of the symptoms commonly associated with food intolerance:

- Colic (in babies)
- Vomiting
- Persistent diarrhoea
- Poor appetite
- Recurrent ear infections
- Asthma
- Stomach aches
- Rash around the mouth
- Rhinitis (runny or congested nose)
- Glue ear
- Eczema
- Urticaria (hives or nettle rash)
- Headaches
- Migraine
- Hyperactivity
- Aching muscles and joints
- Infantile insomnia
- Bedwetting

By feeding your child a fresh, wholesome and varied diet, and following the guidelines in the Avoiding Allergies chart (page 51), you should be able to avoid any problems with food intolerance.

## When to introduce certain foods to help prevent allergies

Allergies seem to be on the rise. Recent figures claim that as many as one in four children under eight now suffers from eczema, one in five has asthma, and one in 200 is allergic to peanuts. Of course this growth is not only due to diet. But the tendency to introduce allergenic foods too early is certainly greatly increasing the risk. My Avoiding Allergies chart (see opposite) shows which foods are safe to introduce when, and takes the anxiety out of weaning.

Signs of an allergic reaction to a food can include:

- Vomiting

- Itching

- Swelling of the lips, throat, tongue, face and head

- Rashes

- Flushing

- Difficulty in breathing

Allergic reactions are not that common but if they do occur, do not give your child the suspected food again for a few weeks. Then, when you reintroduce it, make sure you are not far from your doctor's surgery. Many people are unaware that it is the second exposure to an allergen that results in the worst allergic reaction.

## Does your child have an 'allergic face'? What to look for:

- Runny, congested nose

- Dark rings under eyes

- Creases in the bottom eyelids

- Red ears

- Line across bridge of nose caused by palm of hand being rubbed up the nose to relieve irritation

## Avoiding allergies chart

You can reduce the risk of your child developing allergies by delaying the introduction of the following foods until the ages indicated.

### 6–9 months
Fresh vegetables (except potato, tomato, aubergine, peppers)

Fresh fruits (except citrus and strawberries)

Dried fruits (unsulphured)

Gluten-free grains (rice, millet, quinoa and buckwheat)

Beans and pulses

Organic poultry and meat

Fish* (except shellfish)

### 9–12 months
Gluten grains (oats, rye, barley)
Corn
Potato, tomato, aubergine, peppers

Soya products*

Ground nuts* ground seeds*

### 12–24 months
Wheat (bread, pasta, flour)
Dairy products (whole cow's milk, cheese, yogurt)
Citrus fruit

Eggs*

### 24+ months
Shellfish*
Strawberries*

### 5+ years
Whole nuts*

* The foods marked with an asterisk are those that are most likely to cause an allergic reaction.

You may be surprised to see potatoes, tomatoes, peppers and aubergines amongst the list of foods to avoid until after nine months. The reason for this is that they all belong to a family of foods called *Solanaceae* (better known as the deadly nightshade family). The theory, developed by Dr Norman Childers in the 1970s, is that these foods contain natural toxins which provoke a gradual reaction in susceptible people. In his opinion, arthritis, headaches, depression, diarrhoea, dry mouth and eyes and high blood pressure could all be symptoms of the nightshade toxins.

Tomatoes can be particularly allergenic in babies. I have seen both hyperactivity and eczema provoked by the early consumption of tomatoes. If you are an allergic family, it's best to err on the side of caution and choose from the many other fruits and vegetables available before introducing the above foods to your baby.

## Eating a wheat-free diet

Whether or not your child is intolerant of wheat, it's a good idea not to rely on it too much. There are many alternatives to wheat and wheat products, including:

- Breads, cakes and biscuits made from rye, oats, barley, corn and brown rice

- German rye pumpernickel bread

- Puffed rice cakes and rice crackers

- Rye crispbreads (check ingredients)

- Oat cakes (check ingredients)

- Porridge made from oats, barley, brown rice, buckwheat and millet

- Puffed brown rice cereals, wheat-free muesli and cornflakes

- Barley flour, rye flour, buckwheat flour, potato flour, soya flour, arrowroot flour, cornflour (maize only)

- Rice noodles

- Buckwheat, barley, rice and corn pastas

On pages 55–56 are some suggestions for wheat-free menus, which show how easy it is to give your child a varied, appetising diet without any wheat at all.

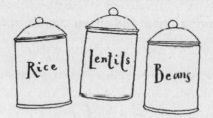

## What about dairy products?

You will notice that, throughout this book, I refer to 'appropriate milk' or talk about dairy alternatives like soya milk, oat milk, rice milk and nut milks. This is because I do not believe in giving babies whole cow's milk or cow's milk products (like yogurt or cheese) until after the age of one, as milk is a common cause of allergy in babies and is extremely mucus-forming. (A more detailed insight into the dairy debate and the calcium question is given in Chapter 5 'One Year and Older'.)

In the meantime, follow the guidelines in each chapter depending on your baby's age and he will experience the health benefits of not being introduced to dairy products too early. This information ranges from alternatives to cow's milk formulas for bottle-feeding to what appropriate milks you can use for a toddler. My children did not have any dairy products at all until the ages of 15–19 months. I then tried them out on organic natural yogurt with a fruit purée and progressed from there to occasional use of grated organic Cheddar cheese in a recipe. Now dairy products are an integral part of their diet and I just make sure that they do not have too much too often.

Alternatives to dairy products include:

- Soya milk, oat milk, rice milk, coconut milk, almond milk

- Dairy-free spreads like soya margarine, Vitaquell and Vitaseig

- Soya yogurt (live, natural and fruit-flavoured are available)

- Soya cheeses (both hard and cream cheeses available)

On pages 57–59 are some suggestions for dairy-free menus.

# Wheat-free menus

## MENU 1

### BREAKFAST
Oat Porridge (page 106) with organic whole milk, soya milk,
or goat's milk
Ryvita with 100 per cent fruit jam
Appropriate milk to drink

### LUNCH
Fishy Rice (page 172) and salad
Fruit Smoothie (page 185)
Water to drink

### TEA
Corn Pasta with Quick and Easy Pasta Sauce (page 136)
Fruit salad and live yogurt
Water to drink

## MENU 2

### BREAKFAST
Puffed rice cereal with banana, raisins, organic whole milk,
soya milk or goat's milk
Gluten-free toast and marmite
Appropriate milk to drink

### LUNCH
Liver Casserole (page 164), mashed potato and broccoli
Baked Apple with Molasses (page 188) and custard
Water to drink

*continues* ▶

### TEA
Nutty Leek, Potato and Parsnip Soup (page 131) with
Oatcake Animals (page 183)
Banana
Water to drink

## MENU 3

### BREAKFAST
Millet Porridge (page 94) with fresh fruit and organic
whole milk,
soya milk or goat's milk
Rice cakes with cashew butter
Appropriate milk to drink

### LUNCH
Lentil Shepherd's pie (page 144) and spring greens
Brown Rice Pudding (page 190)
Water to drink

### TEA
Tuna Pasta Bake (page 169)
Fresh Fruit Juice Jelly (page 192)
Water to drink

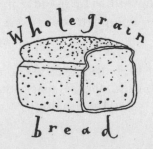

# Dairy-free menus

## MENU 1

### BREAKFAST
Oat Porridge (page 106) with rice milk, chopped banana
and tahini
Wholemeal toast and dairy-free spread with 100 per cent fruit
blackcurrant jam
Soya milk, rice milk, almond milk to drink

### LUNCH
Chicken Stew (page 161) with brown rice, broccoli and carrots
Mango Hedgehog (page 187)
Water or diluted fruit juice to drink

### TEA
Buckwheat Pasta with Quick and Easy Pasta Sauce (page 136)
Soya yogurt
Water or diluted fruit juice to drink

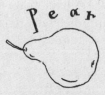

## MENU 2

### BREAKFAST
Tofu Scramble (page 129) with wholemeal toast
Satsuma
Soya milk, rice milk, almond milk to drink

*continues* ►

## LUNCH

Salmon Fishcake (page 173) with Salad Platter (page 158)
Baked Apple with Molasses (page 188) and Custard (page 188),
made with soya milk
Water or diluted fruit juice to drink

## TEA

Immune Boosting Soup (page 133) and rice cake croûtons
Banana Cake (page 200) and pear pieces
Water or diluted fruit juice to drink

## Other dairy-free recipes

Raw Muesli – dairy-free version (page 128)

Boiled Egg and Soldiers

Nutty Leek, Potato and Parsnip Soup (page 131)

Courgette Soup (page 135)

Sunshine Tofu Risotto (page 138)

Vegetable Casserole (page 140)

Herby Millet (page 141)

Bean Stew (page 142)

Lentil Shepherds's Pie (page 144)

Nut Roast (page 143)

Vegetarian Spaghetti Bolognese (page 146)

Potato Cakes (page 149)

Fish Stew (page 175)

Baked Eggs (page 156)

Chinese Stir-fry with Tofu (page 150)

Salmon Pesto Spaghetti (page 174)

Chicken Fingers (page 160)

Classic Lamb Stew (page 163)

Fish Pie – dairy-free version (page 170)

Vegetable Rich Mince (page 166)

Liver Casserole (page 164)

Hearty Winter Stew (page 168)

Chicken Parcels (page 159)

Fishy Rice (page 172)

Instant Fishy Pasta Sauce (page 174)

Gem Squash Surprise (page 167)

Salmon Parcels (page 176)

Baked Sea Bass (page 177)

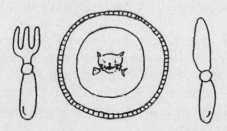

# Organic versus non-organic food

## Should a baby's first food be organic?

Early in 1995 the US Environmental Working Group organised tests to measure the incidence of pesticides in jars of baby food made by Heinz, Beech Nut and Gerber. The tests detected 16 different pesticides, including eight possible cancer promoters, eight that affect brain function and five which disrupt the hormonal system. Two or more pesticides were found in 18 per cent of the samples.

Weight for weight, babies eat far more fruit and vegetables, fruit juices, milk and other pesticide-containing foods than an adult eats. This means that babies may be exceeding the acceptable adult level of pesticide exposure. Many pesticides are known to be carcinogenic (cancer-forming) and, as infancy is a time of rapid development and growth, it is a time of extreme vulnerability. A child's body can also retain a greater portion of a given toxin because their gastrointestinal tract is more easily penetrated.

In addition, organic food may contain many more nutrients than non-organic. Tests carried out by the Camden Food and Drink Association showed that organic potatoes contained 26 per cent more zinc; organic tomatoes 17.5 per cent more vitamin C and 25 per cent more vitamin A; and organic apples 11 per cent more vitamin C.

Weaning babies onto an organic diet is now relatively easy. Most supermarkets have a range of organic vegetables and fruit and the Soil Association publishes a directory called *Where to Buy Organic Food* (see Resources). There is also a large choice of organic baby foods, ranging from organic formula milks to dried and 'wet' weaning foods. Brands include Osska fresh organic babyfoods, Baby Organix, Hipp, Boots Mother's Recipe organic baby food, and Cow and Gate Organic Choice. Many can be bought in supermarkets, chemists or healthfood stores. They are useful as storecupboard supplies or for when you are travelling.

Even if you do not feed your child organically at any other time, six to 12 months is the time to do it. This will avoid unnecessary exposure to pesticides, some of which are known to be carcinogenic. I do, however, feed my family as much organic food as possible. I feel particularly strongly about using organic meat and dairy products. Non-organic animals are not only exposed to pesticides, but also to antibiotics and hormones, residues of which can be detected in the meat or milk. You will find a list of organic suppliers under 'Resources'. One way to reduce the cost of organic food is to eat less meat and use a bigger variety of grains, vegetables and pulses, which are a great deal cheaper.

## Raising a healthy vegetarian child

Vegetarianism is becoming increasingly popular. It is estimated in the UK that 3 per cent of children between the ages of four and 11 are now vegetarian and this is growing year by year. Childhood is a time of tremendous growth and development so it is important to make sure that your children are receiving all the nutrients they require to grow up strong and healthy. It is very easy to be vegetarian; it is not quite so easy to be a really good vegetarian!

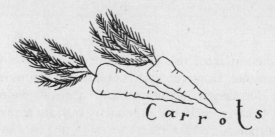

Carrots

| | Foods excluded | Protein source | Nutrients at risk of deficiency |
|---|---|---|---|
| **Lacto-ovo vegetarian** | Red meat<br>Poultry<br>Fish | Milk<br>Cheese<br>Yogurt<br>Eggs<br>Beans and lentils<br>Nuts and seeds<br>Soya products | Energy (kcal)<br>Iron |
| **Lacto vegetarian** | Red meat<br>Poultry<br>Fish<br>Eggs | Milk<br>Cheese<br>Yogurt<br>Beans and lentils<br>Nuts and seeds<br>Soya products | Energy (kcal)<br>Iron<br>Vitamin D |
| **Vegan** | Red meat<br>Poultry<br>Fish<br>Eggs<br>Milk<br>Cheese<br>Yogurt | Beans and lentils<br>Nuts and seeds<br>Soya products<br>Certain grains | Energy (kcal)<br>Iron<br>Protein<br>Vitamins A and D<br>Vitamin B2<br>Vitamin B12<br>Calcium<br>Zinc |

The children at most risk of deficiencies are obviously those on a vegan diet. However, with careful meal planning, a well-balanced diet can be achieved. Some general guidelines for raising a healthy child the vegetarian way are shown in the following chart.

1. If you are vegan, maintain breast-feeding for the first 12 months, after which time fortified soya milks can be added to the diet. This will ensure adequate calcium, vitamin B12 and vitamin D2.

2. The initial process of weaning a vegetarian or vegan baby is the same as for other diets. A wide variety of foods should be introduced, starting with fruit and vegetable purées as well as gluten-free grains like rice and millet.

3. Babies need plenty of energy. Breakfast cereals should be made as a thick porridge, not as a watery gruel. Adding 1 teaspoon flaxseed oil (available at healthfood shops) will increase the calorie content and provide essential fatty acids necessary for brain growth and immune function.

4. Include energy-dense foods such as nut and seed butters, like almond butter and tahini (sesame seed spread), as well as freshly ground nuts and seeds.

5. Offer both pulses and grains for good protein intake. Include grains which are high in protein like quinoa and amaranth.

6. Include soya products like tofu and soya yogurts which are high in calcium and protein. Ensure the source is free of genetically modified soya. All organic soya products are guaranteed GMO-free.

7. Prepare plenty of green leafy vegetables, like broccoli, kale, spinach and watercress, for an adequate intake of magnesium, iron, calcium and folic acid.

8. Include a variety of whole grains, beans and lentils, dried fruits, nut and nut butters, green leafy vegetables and fortified breakfast cereals as good sources of iron. Include

vitamin C-rich foods like citrus fruit, kiwi, berries, blackcurrants or green leafy vegetables in each meal to enhance iron absorption.

9. Use low-salt yeast extracts as a valuable source of B vitamins.

10. Include zinc-rich foods such as seeds, nuts, whole grains and pulses.

11. Use fortified, unhydrogenated margarines like Vitaquell for spreading and extra-virgin olive oil for cooking as sources of fat-soluble vitamins.

12. Include plenty of carrots, tomatoes, peppers, apricots and squashes as sources of beta-carotene, the precursor to vitamin A.

13. Avoid giving tea or excessive amounts of wholewheat cereals and bread which can hinder mineral absorption.

14. Don't let babies and young children fill up on liquids before meals.

15. Whilst breast-feeding, vegan mothers should take a multivitamin and mineral supplement which includes vitamins B2 and D as well as additional calcium, magnesium and zinc.

16. From six months all vegetarian babies should receive vitamin drops which can be mixed in with their food.

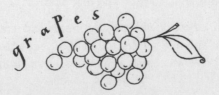

# Unwilling eaters

This is one of the most common reasons why mothers bring their children to see me in my practice. By following the guidelines in this book you should be able to avoid the fussy eating syndrome. However, if a member of your family does develop poor eating habits, here are a few suggestions.

Avoid the trap of repetitive feeding. Many families rotate 7–10 meals that they have regularly week in and week out. But it is important to provide plenty of variety, as limiting your child's diet will limit his nutrient intake and can encourage food intolerance as well as food faddism. Wheat is often included in every meal, either as cereal, bread or pasta. Yet not only is wheat one of the most common food allergens in children but it also contains phytate, which binds with important minerals like calcium, magnesium and zinc and prevents their absorption. Offer wheat-based foods only once a day, and if your child loves pasta (as most children do) introduce other forms of pasta as well. You can now buy corn pasta, rice pasta, barley pasta and buckwheat pasta – all in a variety of shapes and colours. Instead of wheat-based cereals, offer oat porridge, raw muesli, rice cereals or unsugared cornflakes with banana and raisins. Alternatives to bread are rye crackers, rice cakes, oat cakes or gluten-free varieties of bread which can be made into toast.

Avoid the junk food syndrome. Ready-prepared foods may be quick and easy but they are also heavily laden with salt, sugar and unwanted flavour enhancers. Cooking for the family does not need to take an enormous amount of time but it does require mental preparation. Spend a few minutes at the beginning of each week working out the family's meals. After all, baking a cod fillet takes just as little time as cooking a few fish fingers and is an infinitely better choice nutritionally.

Avoid constant snacking. This is often the start of the slippery slope of food faddism. Children grow very fast and require three small meals and a couple of snacks during the day. However, if your child is starting to refuse meals but still snacking then the alarm bells should start ringing. Snacks should be fruit-based: an apple or a fruit and nut bar, a sugar-free muffin or a piece of banana bread; not crisps, chocolate, lollipops, cakes or biscuits. No child will sit down and eat a lovingly prepared healthy meal whilst regularly consuming these snacks, which are high in sugar, salt and saturated fat.

Milk can also often be a culprit in suppressing a child's appetite. Milk in itself is a food rather than just a drink and is incredibly filling. Once your child is over the age of one, he does not need to receive any more than 600 ml (1 pint) of milk or equivalent in dairy products (cheese, yogurt) a day. If your child is drinking more than this and seems to have little appetite, cut down on the milk.

It is not surprising that many children who are picky eaters very often have parents who are picky too! As parents, we need to lead by example. Your children will do what you do and not what you say. Meals are social occasions, so try to sit, eat and talk with your children whenever possible.

If a meal is refused, try not to get angry (often the best tactic is to ignore it). Do not offer any snacks until the next meal, and after a couple of missed meals you should have a hungry child on your hands. In the words of Dr Christopher Green, 'No child has ever starved to death through stubborness.'

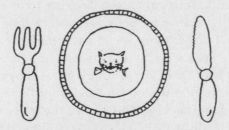

# Making changes

If you have older children who already have established eating patterns which are less than desirable, here are some suggestions on how to make some simple changes for the better by substituting healthier alternatives for some of the worst culprits:

| Culprit | Alternative |
|---|---|
| Ribena and other squashes | 100 per cent fruit concentrates, like apple and blackcurrant |
| Fizzy drinks | Appletize, Aqua Libra |
| Tomato ketchup | Sugar-free varieties, like Whole Earth |
| Cakes and biscuits | Home-made ones (see recipes) |
| Chips | Home-made Chips (page 139) |
| Sweets and chocolates | Fruit bars, lollipops and carob bars, available at healthfood stores. |

## Introduce variety

It's better to concentrate on introducing new, healthier food, rather than just on removing the bad. If your children love pasta, that's fine. But try all the different varieties, rather than just white pasta. You can now buy wholemeal pasta, corn pasta, rice pasta, buckwheat pasta and barley pasta, amongst others. If the only fish your children will eat is fish fingers then introduce home-made Fish Fingers (page 171) and use a wider variety of fish, like cod, haddock, coley and sea bass. Make a big Fish Pie (page 170) and add some mackerel or some prawns and other seafood. Within no time you will have improved the whole family's diet without much resistance.

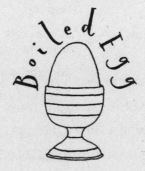

# 2.

# The First Six Months

This chapter explains why I believe
that breast is best and how to look after
yourself whilst breast-feeding. For those
who are unable to breast-feed, I have
also included information on the best
bottle-feeding options.

Having a baby is a truly magical event, and for many people it rates as the happiest moment of their lives. However, once the initial euphoria has passed, the prospect of 'holding the baby', so to speak, can be a bit daunting. This is quite natural and soon passes. One decision that you will probably have made long before the birth is whether you are going to breast-feed or bottle-feed. The best piece of advice I was ever given on this subject came from a great friend, a nurse, who, whilst I was pregnant, told me not to think about the 'what if's' but to assume that I would be able to breast-feed, as it was the most natural thing in the world. My baby would need feeding and I had the food. It sounds rather simplistic but it did take away the anxiety that not just I, but a lot of expectant mothers feel, especially as we all tend to read far too many baby books when we are pregnant and then worry about all the things that could go wrong!

This chapter explains why I believe that breast is best and how to look after yourself whilst breast-feeding. For those who are unable to breast-feed, I have also included information on the best bottle-feeding options.

## Why breast really is best

Breast milk is a perfectly balanced food that will provide your baby with all the nourishment he needs for the first few months. Being a new mother can be exhausting, and one of the blessings of breast-feeding is that it requires no preparation; you don't need any special equipment and the milk is always at exactly the right temperature. Furthermore, breast milk contains special substances uniquely designed to protect your baby from infection and enhance his overall defences by helping his immune system to mature. It will also protect a baby susceptible to allergies due to its high level of essential fatty acids (deficient in most formula milks).

Breast-feeding, like any new skill, can take time to master. But the benefits far outweigh any problems you may encounter early on. Ideally your baby should be put to your breast very soon after the birth, as it is at this time that his sucking instinct is strongest. However, don't be alarmed if your baby does not feed straight away. Some babies are exhausted by the birth and need to catch up on a little sleep before a feed. During these first few days, you will produce a substance called colostrum rather than milk. It is not produced in great quantity but it is rich in protein, vitamins and minerals, as well as the antibodies which will protect your baby from infection and help to build his immune system. These substances are also anti-allergenic and they cannot be duplicated in formula milks.

During this time it is important not to let your baby suckle endlessly at the breast, as this may cause soreness. When your baby latches on, he needs to open his mouth wide and take in not only the nipple but also much of the coloured area underneath the nipple (the areola). This takes practice for both of you and you may have to keep trying. If you feel that your baby is not latching on properly, slip your little finger gently into the corner of his mouth to release the suction, and try again. Although this can be tiring, it will help to prevent sore and cracked nipples and will also encourage your baby to latch on properly without getting into bad habits early on. If you need more help or would like to talk to someone about breast-feeding, do talk to your health visitor or local breast-feeding counsellor (see Resources).

## How long should I breast-feed?

This appears to be a controversial topic at the moment. Some mothers breast-feed until their children are five years old and others only for four months. In order to provide optimum nutrition for your baby, it's best to breast-feed exclusively for six months. After this time, with the inclusion of solid food, I recommend that you supplementary breast-feed until they are a year old. If you are back at work after four months, then a morning and night-time breast-feed will still be beneficial. Breast-feeding for longer than a year has more to do with comfort and the mother/child bond than nutritional content and so it is entirely a question of personal choice.

## The better breast-feeding diet

Remember that the quality of your breast milk depends to a certain extent on the quality of your diet. So here are some tips on how to look after yourself whilst breast-feeding:

- Eat three meals and two good snacks a day. Listen to your body and eat when you are hungry. Breast-feeding increases your appetite.

- Drink at least 1.5 litres (2½ pints) of filtered tap water or mineral water a day. Always have a drink beside you when you sit down to feed, as the baby suckling will stimulate a thirst and there is nothing more annoying than wanting a drink when you have just got settled.

- Eat at least five portions of fruit and vegetables a day (preferably organic).

- Snack on fruit, nuts and seeds, rather than sugary snacks.

- Eat plenty of high-fibre foods like wholemeal bread, oats, brown rice, pulses, fruit and vegetables.

- Eat oily fish at least twice a week; mackerel, salmon, herring, pilchard, sardine and fresh tuna are all good sources of essential fatty acids for you and your baby.

- An excellent high-protein and essential fatty acid drink, ideal for breakfast or when you are just too tired to eat, is an Energy Shake (page 209). It is quick and easy and quite delicious.

- Take a good-quality vitamin and mineral supplement to boost your own vital body stores. Some companies produce special formulas for lactating mums (see Resources). This supplement should include:

| | |
|---|---|
| Beta-carotene | 5000 iu |
| B complex: | B1 10 mg |
| | B2 10 mg |
| | B3 100 mg |
| | B5 100 mg |
| | B6 20 mg |
| | B12 10 mcg |
| | Folic acid 400 mcg |
| | Biotin 200 mcg |
| Vitamin C | 1000 mg |
| Vitamin D | 400 iu |
| Vitamin E | 100 iu |
| Calcium | 600 mg |
| Magnesium | 300 mg |
| Iron | 15 mg |
| Zinc | 25 mg |
| Selenium | 100 mcg |
| Chromium | 100 mcg |

You may find that you need to use a combination of supplements to achieve these levels e.g. a multivitamin and mineral, a 1000 mg tablet of vitamin C and a couple of calcium and magnesium tablets. (See Resources for good suppliers.)

# Things to avoid when you are breast-feeding

As well as making sure that your diet contains all the nutrients that are good for your baby, it is also important to avoid the substances that are known to be detrimental and can be passed on to him through breast milk. Here are the most important ones:

- Caffeine (found in coffee, tea, chocolate, coca cola and other fizzy drinks) is a drug to which the body can become addicted. It can cause irritability and sleeplessness in your baby as well as you.

- Theobromine, found in chocolate, is a stimulant that can make your baby irritable – rather like caffeine.

- Nicotine, found in cigarettes, can affect your baby's heart rate and cause vomiting and diarrhoea.

- Alcohol can damage your baby's brain cells. Drink diluted fruit juices, Appletize, Aqua Libra or fizzy water instead. If you do have an occasional drink, enjoy it during the last feed of the day and avoid breast-feeding for at least four hours.

- Artificial sweeteners like aspartame (found in fizzy drinks, squashes and low-calorie foods) can make your baby hyperactive.

- Avoid dieting whilst you are breast-feeding. Your fat stores contain residues of pesticides from food that you have eaten through your life; dramatic weight loss releases these stored toxins into your blood, from where they can easily be transmitted to breast milk. If you eat healthily, you will find that you gradually lose weight during breast-feeding in any case.

- Avoid over-the-counter as well as prescription drugs whilst breast-feeding, as these can affect your baby's development. If you take any regular medication, consult your doctor regarding breast-feeding.

# Bottle-feeding

Although breast milk is the perfect food for your infant, not all women are able to breast-feed their babies and so a suitable formula must be found. Until a baby is a year old, it must be fed either breast milk or formula milk. Whole cow's milk, carton soya milks or whole goat's milk are unmodified and are therefore unsuitable.

There are, however, a number of specially designed formulas which are suitable for bottle-feeding your newborn which I have discussed in preferential order. They have been formulated to be as close to human milk as possible.

## Goat's milk infant formula

Formulas made from goat's milk tend to be less allergenic than cow's milk formulas. They are suitable from birth and are more digestible than cow's milk formulas as they form smaller, softer curds in the stomach, making it easier for your baby's immature digestive system to cope. Goat's milk formulas can often be tolerated by babies sensitive to cow's milk formulas as the gamma- casein present in cow's milk is absent from goat's milk. The leading goat's milk formula, 'Nanny', also has a good essential fatty acid content and is my number one choice of formula (see Resources).

## Cow's milk infant formula

This type of formula milk is the most commonly used by parents who are bottle-feeding their babies. There are three main types of cow's milk formula: whey-dominant, casein-dominant, and follow-on formula milks. Whey is the clear liquid left after the milk protein has clotted (as in cheese-making). Whey-based formulas are usually given to newborn babies, as the ratio of casein to whey is closer to that of breast milk, and whey is supposed to be easier to digest. Casein-dominant and follow-on formulas are for bottle-fed babies over six months. They are denser milks for hungrier babies and also contain added iron.

### Common brands of cow's milk infant formulas

Babynat is my first choice but the others do not appear in order of preference.

Babynat
Cow and Gate Premium
Farley's First Milk
Sainsbury's First Menu: First Stage
Milupa Aptamil
SMA Gold
Boots Formula 1

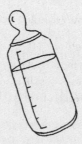

'Babynat' is imported from France. It contains essential fatty acids, which many of the other cow's milk formulas do not, and it is produced from organic cattle – which is a bonus.

## Soya-based formula

I'm not a great fan of soya-based formulas and therefore do not recommend using them. However, they are an obvious choice for an infant with lactose intolerance and these formulas are also the only option for vegan mothers who are not breast-feeding. However, they do have a relatively high allergenicity. And, since they are free of lactose (milk sugar), they are sweetened with glucose syrup or other sugary agents which are implicated as a major cause of tooth decay. Another cause for concern is the presence of phytoestrogens, as these can behave like a weak form of the female hormone oestrogen. There is a worry that the level of phytoestrogens in the formula may affect the hormonal balance of the baby. Research is underway to establish any link and until any concrete evidence is revealed, these formulas are still available. Some of them may contain undesirable levels of aluminium and, for this reason, soya formulas are not recommended for premature babies or those suffering from kidney problems.

> **Marks out of 10**
>
> This is how I would rank the various options.
>
> Breast-feeding: 10
> Goat's milk formula: 7
> Organic cow's milk formula: 6
> Soya formula: 4

## Tips on bottle-feeding

- If you use tap water for your formula feeds, make sure you only boil the water in the kettle once. Re-boiling will increase the sodium content of the water which can be dangerous for your baby's health.

- If, whilst abroad, you use boiled bottled water to make up your formula feeds, watch out for mineral levels which can vary. Only bottled water with a sodium content of less than 10 mg per 100 ml (4 fl oz) should be used.

- Bottle-fed babies do get thirsty. Offer warm, bottled water twice a day, or more often in very hot weather.

- Ensure adequate omega 6 and omega 3 essential fatty acids intake (see pages 6–8 for a full description of these 'good fats'). Omega 6 can be administered by rubbing the oil from a 500 mg capsule of evening primrose oil onto your baby's tummy or inside thighs once a day. It will be absorbed through the skin and can help to prevent skin problems like eczema. Never give a capsule orally, as this can cause choking. Omega 3 essential fatty acids can be added to the formula in the form of flaxseed oil. A few drops can be added to each bottle, after heating, to total no more than 1 teaspoon in a 24-hour period (see Resources for suppliers). Breast-fed babies receive all the essential fatty acids they need from breast milk.

• Once a day, add a quarter of a teaspoon of Bifidobacterium Infantis (see Resources) to the milk just before feeding. These beneficial bacteria are prevalent in breast-fed babies and lacking in bottle-fed babies. They will help to protect your baby against tummy bugs. (Do not heat the milk with the Bifidobacterium Infantis – if you do so you will destroy the beneficial bacteria.)

## Does a breast-fed baby need bottles?

Babies who are breast-fed do not, in theory, require any extra liquid. However, in practice, you may find it very useful to introduce bottles of warm, boiled water every other day from two weeks after the birth. It is unlikely that your baby will want any, but by offering him a bottle you are introducing him to the feel of a plastic teat which may make changing from breast to bottle much easier later on.

You also then have the added advantage of being able to express some breast milk and allowing someone else to feed your baby. Many mothers prefer to breast feed exclusively and then introduce a feeder cup at around eight months. But if you are going back to work I would recommend introducing bottles, since they will inevitably become a part of your baby's life.

# 3.

# Six to Nine Months – First Foods

At around six months your baby will be
ready to enjoy his first solid food. Start
with tiny tastes of vegetable and fruit purées.
By introducing new foods one at a time
you will be able to notice any reaction to the
food. In this chapter you will find recipes for
both cooked and raw purées.

Aт AROUND SIX MONTHS your baby will be ready to enjoy his first tastes of fruit and vegetable purées. It is important not to introduce solids too early, as this will put a strain on your baby's immature digestive system. It will also increase the risk of allergies since, whilst developing, your baby's intestinal tract is porous and therefore cannot screen out the big molecules that can cause allergies.

Although British government guidelines recommend that you start weaning after only four months, some paediatricians in America now advocate leaving it until six months and I agree with them. Certainly if there is a history of allergy in your family then exclusively breastfeeding for the first six months is the ideal, as this will reduce your baby's susceptibility. However, it is advisable not to leave weaning much later than six months as by this time an infant's energy requirement is higher. Also vital birth stores of nutrients such as iron and zinc are likely to be running low and will need to be supplied through the diet.

## Introducing solids

When you start your baby on solids, arm yourself with a weaning spoon (available from most chemists) and use a small plastic weaning bowl or the top from one of your baby's bottles (if you are using them). Start your baby with tiny tastes of vegetable and fruit purées. Introduce one food at a time and repeat for two or three days so that you can notice any reaction that your baby may have to the food.

I have found that lunchtime is the best meal to introduce solids for the first time. If you are breastfeeding, allow your baby to start a milk feed before offering any purée. This will stave off any initial hunger or thirst and will avoid him getting angry at you or the spoon. Offer a couple of tastes of the purée and then finish off the milk feed. If you are bottle-feeding, the same rules apply. You may find that at the beginning your baby fusses at the spoon, as it is a new experience. However, it will not take long for him to get the knack, especially at this age, and he will quickly progress onto several teaspoons at mealtimes.

Keeping a food diary is an ideal way to keep track of foods being introduced and is also a lovely memento to keep. A couple of weeks after introducing food for the first time, you can introduce it at breakfast, and then again, after a couple of weeks, at teatime. By seven months, your baby will be on three meals a day. But it is important, at this stage, not to reduce your baby's milk feeds, as the solids are not nutritionally adequate on their own. By week seven, you can introduce food as the first part of lunch and then top up with a milk feed. And by eight months (at week 9 on the weaning chart) you can do the same at teatime. In this way, you will gradually be reducing the breast milk or formula intake, as solid food takes over in terms of bulk and nutritional content. Look at the chart below which sets out the weaning process, week by week, to help you plan your baby's meals.

As I explained in Chapter 1 (page 24), the ice cube method is ideal during the weaning process. At the beginning you can defrost just one ice cube and you will not be wasting additional purée. Remember that every baby's appetite will vary and therefore the quantities I mention in the chart are there only as a rough guide.

If a food can be given raw then give it raw (e.g. mashed banana, avocado, paw paw or very ripe pear). Raw foods of this nature are a wonderful source of vitamins, minerals, water, enzymes and fibre. In this chapter you will find recipes for both cooked and raw purées.

## WEANING CHART

| | Week 1 and 2 | Week 3 and 4 | Week 5 and 6 |
|---|---|---|---|
| **Early morning**<br>e.g.<br>5.30–6.30am | Feed | Feed | – |
| **Breakfast**<br>e.g.<br>8.30–9.30am | Feed<br><br><br>Feed | Feed<br>1–2 teaspoons<br>solids<br>Feed | Feed<br>2–3 teaspoons<br>solids<br>Feed |
| **Lunchtime**<br>e.g.<br>11.30–12.30pm | Feed<br>1–2 teaspoons<br>solids<br>Feed | Feed<br>3–4 teaspoons<br>solids<br>Feed | Feed<br>5–6 teaspoons<br>solids<br>Feed |
| **Teatime**<br>e.g.<br>3.30–4.30pm | Feed | Feed<br><br><br>Feed | Feed<br>2–3 teaspoons<br>solids<br>Feed |
| **Bedtime**<br>e.g.<br>6.30–7.30pm | Feed | Feed | Feed |
| **Comments** | At lunch introduce small tastes of fruit or vegetable purée halfway through the breast- or bottle-feed. | Introduce solid food at breakfast halfway through the feed. Increase the amount of solid food at lunchtime, depending on your baby's appetite. All amounts are only guidelines. | Introduce solid food at teatime halfway through the feed A few days later you can introduce two courses at lunchtime, e.g. 2–3 teaspoons of a savoury purée followed by 2–3 teaspoons of fruit purée. |

| Week 7 and 8 | Week 9 and 10 | Week 11 and 12 |
|---|---|---|
| – | – | – |
| Feed<br>1–2 dessertspoons<br>solids<br>Feed | Feed<br>3–4 dessertspoons<br>solids | Feed<br>4–5 dessertspoons<br>solids |
| –<br>4–5 dessertspoons<br>solids<br>Feed | –<br>4–5 dessertspoons<br>solids | –<br>4–5 dessertspoons<br>solids<br>Beaker |
| Feed<br>3–4 dessertspoons<br>solids<br>Feed | –<br>4–5 dessertspoons<br>solids<br>Feed | –<br>4–5 dessertspoons<br>solids<br>Beaker |
| Feed | Feed | Feed |
| Offer solid food as the first part of lunch now and top up with breast or bottle after. Increase the amounts of solid food depending on your baby's appetite. | After lunch offer formula or water from a beaker instead of a feed. Offer solid food as first part of tea. Your baby may be able to handle a beaker for himself from 8–10 months. | Offer a beaker at teatime. |

## Iron-rich foods as first foods

Once past six months, your baby's iron stores from birth will start to run out, so you need to include good sources of iron in his diet. The iron is important for brain development and it also helps him build up resistance to infection. Iron-deficiency (or anaemia) is quite common in toddlers but is easily prevented. At this early weaning stage (six months) you will be feeding your baby only on vegetables, fruit and a few grains, so here is a list of good sources of iron which you should be including in his diet:

- Green leafy vegetables (including broccoli, green cabbage, kale, spinach, beetroot tops, watercress, parsley and peas)
- Dried fruit purées (made from unsulphured dried fruit)
- Whole lentils (boiled)
- Crude blackstrap molasses
- Whole grains (like millet and amaranth)
- Iron-fortified baby cereals (e.g. rice-based varieties)

Feeding your baby with foods which are rich in vitamin C at the same meal will greatly increase the iron absorption from these plant foods. Examples of good vitamin C sources you can include in your baby's diet at this stage are: all green leafy vegetables, kiwi fruit, blackcurrants, papaya and mango.

## Enjoy, enjoy!

Introducing solid food to a baby is great fun. It is so exciting watching them experiencing new smells, tastes and textures. This stage passes really quickly, so enjoy it while it lasts.

If your baby doesn't like a certain taste or texture, don't be alarmed; try other foods, rather than persisting with an unpopular one. Babies have preferences, just like adults!

# Recipes for six to nine months

This recipe section is divided into cooked purées and raw food purées suitable as your baby's first foods. As you can see, most are made in bulk to freeze using the ice cube method (see page 24). I have only included single fruit and vegetable recipes to get you started but all those below can be mixed and matched together. For example, you can defrost two different vegetable purées to make a double vegetable purée. The variations are endless; experiment with your baby's tastebuds and discover his favourites.

Avoid introducing all the very sweet fruits and vegetables at the beginning – ring the changes so that your baby develops a taste for all vegetables. Remember variety is the key and will encourage your baby to have an adventurous appetite in toddlerhood. When preparing your baby's first purées it is important to make them really smooth in texture as some babies do gag on the tiniest lump. Once they are used to the sensation of eating solids, coarser purées are fine.

An asterisk* indicates that the recipe can be frozen.

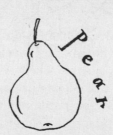

# Carrot Purée*

Carrot is a marvellous first food for your baby. It is naturally sweet, smooth in texture and rich in beta-carotene, the plant form of vitamin A, which is a potent antioxidant.

**MAKES ABOUT 21 CUBES**

- a 450 g (1lb) bag of organic carrots
- 150 ml (5 fl oz) filtered water

Peel, top and tail and slice the carrots. Put them in a pan with the water, bring to the boil and simmer for 10–15 minutes until soft. Alternatively, you can steam them to retain more of the nutrients. It just takes a little longer. Purée the carrot using some of the cooking water until you get your desired consistency.

At eight months you can try your baby out on very finely grated raw carrot. It retains all its vitamins and natural sweetness and is a good way to encourage him to eat raw foods. Grated carrot in a salad won't seem such an alien food at a later age! For an older child, raw carrots are a brilliant natural cure for constipation, as they are rich in fibre.

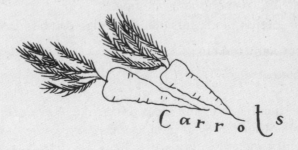

Carrots

# Apple Purée*

Apple purée is another popular first purée and mixes well with other fruit and vegetable purées. Apples can be a good source of vitamin C and apple purée is a traditional healing food for a baby with diarrhoea.

**MAKES ABOUT 30 CUBES**

a 1 kg (2 lb) bag of organic eating apples, peeled and cored
250 ml (9 fl oz) filtered water

Put the apples in a pan with the water, bring to the boil and simmer until soft. Purée to your desired consistency.

To add variety of flavour, add a couple of pinches of ground cinnamon when you cook the apple.

# Butternut Squash Purée*

Butternut squash is rather like a pumpkin but tubular in shape. It is easily digested and rarely causes allergies, which makes it an excellent weaning food. Like other orange fruits and vegetables, it is rich in beta-carotene.

**MAKES ABOUT 28 CUBES**

1 butternut squash

Cut the squash in half and remove the seeds. Peel and chop up the flesh. Steam for 8–10 minutes until soft. Purée to desired consistency and freeze the excess.

# Sweet Potato Purée*

Another delicious first purée, providing good sources of potassium, vitamin C, fibre and beta-carotene. Sweet potatoes make an excellent alternative to potatoes during the early stages of weaning.

**MAKES ABOUT 35 CUBES**

1 kg (2lb) sweet potatoes
filtered water

Peel, wash and chop the sweet potatoes. Add enough filtered water to cover, bring to the boil and simmer for 20–30 minutes until soft. Alternatively, you can steam it to retain more of its nutrients. Mash or purée to desired consistency.

## Quick tip
You can just as easily bake a sweet potato. Cook for 45–60 minutes, at 220°C/425°F/Gas Mark 7, scoop out the flesh from the skins and mash with a little boiled water, breast milk or formula.

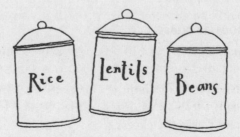

# Broccoli Purée*

Broccoli mixes well with sweet and starchy vegetables like sweet potato, carrot, butternut squash, swede and parsnip. It is also an excellent source of vitamin C and contains useful amounts of folic acid and iron.

### MAKES ABOUT 24 CUBES

a 450 g (1lb) head of organic broccoli
200 ml (7 fl oz) filtered water

Wash the broccoli carefully and cut into florets. Steam, or simmer in the filtered water for 10–15 minutes, until the stalks are soft. Purée to desired consistency and freeze the excess.

# Brown Rice Purée*

This can be as quick and easy as shop-bought baby rice but much healthier.

### MAKES ABOUT 24 CUBES

100 g (4 oz) brown rice
600 ml (1 pint) filtered water

Wash the rice well and place in a pan with the water. Bring to the boil, then gently simmer for 35–40 minutes until the rice is soft and cooked through. Drain the rice in a sieve and purée to your desired consistency. Add some boiled water if the purée is too thick.

This recipe can easily be made in double or triple quantities and frozen using the ice cube method (page 24). It can then be used in both savoury and sweet recipes.

# Date Purée*

This purée is a wonderful all-rounder. It can be added to fresh fruit purées as a pudding, used as a sweetener instead of sugar in baking, and for an older baby it is delicious thinly spread on toast or rice cakes. But do remember that it is a concentrated form of sweetener and should be used sparingly.

### MAKES ABOUT 16 CUBES

250 g (9 oz) pitted dates (not sugar-rolled)
250 ml (9 fl oz) filtered water

Place the dates in a saucepan and pour over the water. Heat gently for 10 minutes, mashing and stirring all the time until soft. Blend to a smooth purée.

Rather than freezing this purée, I prefer to store it in the fridge in a jar for up to two weeks. This means I can use it for other recipes as well.

# Dried Apricot Purée*

Apricot purée is another delicious accompaniment to any of the cereal dishes. Alternatively, it can be mixed with other fresh fruit purées as a pudding. However, I wouldn't encourage you to give it to a baby 'neat' as it is incredibly sweet!

If the apricots are unsulphured they will be dark brown, not bright orange.

### MAKES ABOUT 32 CUBES

a 450 g (1lb) packet of dried, unsulphured apricots
filtered water

Wash the apricots, cover them with boiling filtered water and leave to soak for several hours.

Transfer the water and the apricots to a pan and simmer for 30 minutes until very tender. Then liquidise the apricots and the water to form a smooth purée.

Freeze using the ice cube method (page 24). You will find that they will remain very sticky in the freezer. This is fine – just messy to handle! Alternatively, this purée will keep well in the fridge.

# The best of the 'raw' bunch

Raw food purées are ideal for serving to your baby from an early age. Raw foods are a great source of vitamins, minerals, water and fibre, and they are quick and easy to prepare. These recipes are best served fresh and are not suitable for freezing. They are therefore all based on one serving for a baby.

## Avocado purée

Mash or purée half an avocado and serve immediately. This purée will not keep, as the avocado will turn brown.

## Banana purée

Mash or purée 1 small or ½ large banana and serve immediately. This purée will not keep, as the banana will turn brown.

## Pear purée

Peel and core a very ripe pear. Mash or purée to desired consistency and serve immediately.

## Paw paw (papaya) purée

Slice the paw paw in half and remove the seeds. Scoop out the flesh and mash or purée ½ paw paw and serve immediately.

## Mango purée

Slice off ½ mango and purée the orange flesh. If you have an older child you can slice off the other half and make a Mango Hedgehog (page 187) or a Fruit Smoothie (page 185).

# Banana and Kiwi Fruit Purée

Kiwi fruit are the best source of vitamin C for this age group.

1 small ripe kiwi fruit
1 small ripe banana

Cut the kiwi in half and scoop out the flesh. Blend together with the banana to desired consistency.

# Banana and Melon Purée

A lovely summer purée, rich in beta-carotene, vitamin C and potassium.

¼ small cantaloupe melon
1 small ripe banana

Halve the melon and remove the seeds. Cut into quarters and scoop out the flesh. Blend to a purée with the banana.

# Avocado and Banana Purée

This is, in my opinion, the ultimate purée, packed full of nutrients and quite delicious. Both my children adored this mixture. I have found it especially useful when travelling as you can easily carry around a banana and an avocado and prepare it on the spot.

½ ripe avocado
½ ripe banana

Blend or mash the avocado and banana together and serve immediately.

# Avocado and Beetroot Purée

I do remember the raised eyebrows I used to get when I produced this for my children. It is likely that the beetroot will come out of your baby the same colour as it went in. Please do not be alarmed – this is quite natural! (You can now buy ready-cooked organic beetroot packaged in water, with no added ingredients or preservatives.)

½ ripe avocado
1 small beetroot

Mash the avocado and beetroot together or blend in a food processor and serve immediately.

## Other ideas for first food purées

Peaches, nectarines, plums, fresh apricots, kiwi, melon, unsulphured dried fruits, French beans, mange tout, pumpkin and other squashes, spinach, watercress, cabbage, kale, jerusalem artichoke, parsnip, swede, turnip, lettuce, sweetcorn, celeriac, courgettes, cauliflower, fennel, kohlrabi, peas . . . and many more!

# First breakfasts

## Millet Porridge with Fruit Purée

This is a cheap and nutritious home-made baby breakfast. Millet is a gluten-free grain and therefore an excellent first food for a baby. It is particularly rich in iron, potassium and magnesium as well as being high in protein. To make the porridge really smooth, grind the millet flakes to a powder in a food processor or coffee grinder prior to cooking, and store in an airtight container.

  1 tablespoon millet flakes or ground millet flakes
  150 ml (5 fl oz) breast milk, formula or filtered water
  1 ice cube of fruit purée

In a saucepan mix the millet with the milk or water, a little at a time. Bring to the boil and simmer, stirring, for 12–15 minutes until it thickens. You may have to add some more milk or water if it gets too thick.

Add a cube of fruit purée from the freezer. The advantage of doing this is that it cools the porridge down very fast as it melts. Check the temperature and serve.

# Rice Porridge and Apple and Cinnamon Purée

This is a variation on the millet porridge theme. Rice is also a low-allergenic, gluten-free grain, which is why it has traditionally been served as a first weaning food. In this recipe I have used brown rice rather than the commercially produced white baby rice sold in packets. The packet baby rice reminds me of wallpaper paste – if you need convincing, just taste the stuff! My eldest used to adore this breakfast as a baby. If you buy a large packet of brown rice flakes from a healthfood shop and grind them to a fine powder in a food processor or coffee grinder you can then store the powder in an airtight jar for several weeks.

1 tablespoon ground brown rice flakes
150 ml (5 fl oz) breast milk, formula or filtered water
1 ice cube of Apple and Cinnamon Purée (page 87) or any
alternative fruit purée

Mix the ground brown rice flakes with a little milk or water in a saucepan until you get a creamy consistency. Add the rest of the milk slowly, to prevent lumps forming, and heat gently for 5–10 minutes until cooked. You may need to add a little more milk or water if the porridge thickens too quickly.

Add a cube of Apple and Cinnamon Purée from the freezer and melt the cube in the porridge. Check the temperature and serve.

---

**Quick tip**

You could also use Brown Rice Purée (page 89) for this recipe if you were in a hurry.

---

# First savoury purées

## Chicken Stock Purée*

This makes an excellent first protein purée. It can either be frozen or used as stock for other recipes. Always use an organic chicken carcass.

**MAKES ABOUT 1.3 LITRES (2½ PINTS)**

1 organic chicken carcass (with a little chicken still on it)
2 large carrots, chopped into large chunks
2 medium onions, chopped into quarters
1 head of celery, chopped
1 bouquet garni
1.75 litres (3 pints) filtered water

Put the chicken carcass in a large stainless steel pan. Throw in the vegetables and the bouquet garni and cover with the water. Bring to the boil, cover and simmer for 2 hours. Remove all the bones, allow to cool slightly and liquidise the stock, vegetables and remaining chicken bits.

Freeze in ice cubes, to serve as a savoury purée or to add to other vegetable purées; or freeze in containers as stock for family soups.

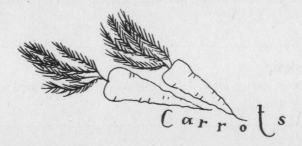

Carrots

# Lentil Purée*

Red lentils are the quickest and easiest of the pulses to cook with and make delicious purées and soups. They are also a useful source of iron.

**MAKES ABOUT 18 CUBES**

1 small leek, washed and finely chopped
1 small carrot, peeled and finely chopped
1 stick of celery, finely chopped
1 teaspoon extra-virgin olive oil
50 g (2 oz) red lentils, washed
300 ml (10 fl oz) filtered water

Sauté the leek, carrot and celery in a little oil for 10 minutes. Add the red lentils and the water and cook gently for 15–20 minutes until the lentils are soft. If the mixture is too thick you can thin it down with a little water or appropriate milk.

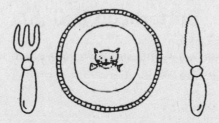

# Cod with Brown Rice and Spinach*

This is an excellent way of introducing babies to fish. You could either freeze it as ice cubes or in larger portions for a hungrier baby.

**MAKES ABOUT 18 CUBES**

1 small boneless and skinless fillet of cod
2 large handfuls of baby spinach
100 ml (4 fl oz) filtered water
50 g (2 oz) brown rice, well cooked

Preheat the oven to 180°C/350°F/Gas Mark 4. Put the cod and the spinach in an oven dish, add the water, cover and bake for 20–30 minutes until cooked. Alternatively you could steam the fish and spinach. Put the fish, spinach and water in a food processor with the cooked rice and blend to desired consistency.

# Butterbean Delight

Butterbeans make a wonderfully creamy purée which is very suitable for a young palate.

**MAKES 1–2 SERVINGS**

white of a small leek, finely chopped
1 teaspoon extra-virgin olive oil
1 small parsnip, peeled and cubed
2 tablespoons tinned cooked butterbeans (no sugar, no salt)
1 teaspoon chopped parsley
150 ml (5 fl oz) filtered water

Sauté the leek in the olive oil for a few minutes until soft. Add the rest of the ingredients and simmer for 20 minutes until the vegetables are cooked. Purée to desired consistency.

# Organic Lamb and Root Veggies*

This delicious combination will help to keep your baby cold-free since garlic is both anti-bacterial and anti-viral.

### MAKES 1–2 SERVINGS

1 clove of garlic, peeled
1 organic lamb cutlet
¼ of a small swede, peeled and chopped

Press the garlic onto the lamb chop and grill for 20 minutes, turning once, until well cooked and the juices run clear. Meanwhile, steam the swede until soft.

Remove the lamb from the bone and purée, along with the swede and a little of the swede water to desired consistency. This could be prepared in bulk for the freezer or could equally be made with some leftover meat from a roast. Any sweet root vegetable will make a nice combination.

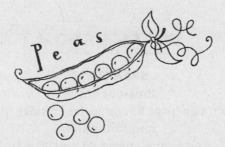

# Sample menus for six to nine months

## WEEKS 1 AND 2

### BREAKFAST
Breast or bottle

### LUNCH
Breast or bottle
Single vegetable purée (see recipes, pages 86–89)

### TEA
Breast or bottle

### BEDTIME
Breast or bottle

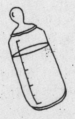

## WEEKS 3 AND 4

### BREAKFAST
Breast or bottle
Rice porridge (page 95) or Millet Porridge (page 94)
and fruit purée
(see recipes, pages 87 and 90–93)

### LUNCH
Breast or bottle
Double vegetable purée (see recipes, pages 86–89)

### TEA
Breast or bottle

### BEDTIME
Breast or bottle

## Sample menus for six to nine months

## WEEKS 5 AND 6

### BREAKFAST
Breast or bottle
Rice Porridge (page 95) or Millet Porridge (page 94)
with fruit purée (see recipes,
pages 87 and 90–93)

### LUNCH
Breast or bottle
Savoury purée followed by fruit purée (see recipes,
pages 87–93)

### TEA
Breast or bottle
Double vegetable purée (see recipes, pages 86–89)

### BEDTIME
Breast or bottle

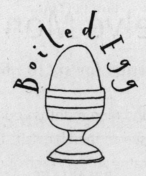

# 4.

# Nine to
# Twelve Months

From around nine months your baby will
show a desire to feed himself. This can be
a fun but rather messy time and a degree
of patience is needed. Invest in a PVC
'splat mat' to catch the mess on the floor
and allow your baby to practise his technique
with one spoon while you continue to
feed him with another.

Having followed the weaning chart, your baby will now be on three meals a day. Solid food will take over as his primary source of nutrition and dietary bulk, with his milk feeds being used as top-ups. Until he reaches a year he still needs to receive 600 ml (1 pint) of formula or breast milk either as a drink or in cooking and you may find that it suits you both to have this mainly at breakfast time and bedtime. However, there is no hard and fast rule, so go with your baby's flow! Start introducing a feeder cup at mealtimes with formula or water in it. Most babies get the hang of using a cup somewhere between eight and ten months.

## Texture

Your baby is now likely to have several teeth and you may find that you can mash his food rather than purée it. This will depend on his temperament as well as his textural likes and dislikes! You can now introduce finger foods and teething rusks. Useful healthy options are: mini rice cakes (which hold together nicely), chunky carrot sticks or apple slices. Do not leave your baby unattended in case of choking.

## Finger foods

From around nine months your baby will show a desire to feed himself. This can be a fun but rather messy time and a degree of patience is needed. Invest in a PVC 'splat mat' to catch the mess on the floor and allow your baby to practise his technique with one spoon while you continue to feed him with another. This will keep you both happy! Introduce finger foods such as raw fruit and vegetables, pieces of cooked chicken, rice cakes and oat fingers (plain or spread with nut butters, seed butters or 100 per cent fruit spreads).

## How much will my baby eat?

Babies between nine and twelve months will, on average, be eating 3–6 tablespoons of food at each meal, divided into a savoury purée followed by a fruit pudding. Remember that this is only to give you an idea of quantities. Every baby's appetite is different.

## What to avoid

Foods to continue avoiding are wheat and milk products, citrus fruits and whole egg, as well as shellfish and whole nuts. To remind yourself, look back at the Avoiding Allergies chart (page 51).

Be particularly vigilant when you introduce ground nuts and seeds for the first time. Introduce the least allergenic first – for example, ground almonds and ground sunflower seeds (or butters made from these) and leave peanut butter until last. As I explained in Chapter 1, you should use only a very little on first and second exposures.

# Recipes for nine to twelve months

Many of the recipes for family meals in Chapter 5 can be adapted for a baby of this age but it is important to check the ingredients against the Avoiding Allergies chart (pages 51) just to make sure. If, on the other hand, you only have one little mouth to feed, here are some quick ideas.

For those who are still breast-feeding and do not want to express milk for the recipes, water or rice milk are adequate substitutes. However, they are not adequate drinking substitutes. A baby of this age still needs to be receiving breast milk or formula, either as a drink or in food, equivalent to 600 ml (1 pint) a day. All serving sizes in this section are based on a baby's portion. An asterisk after the recipe title indicates that the recipe can be frozen.

# Oat Porridge

There is nothing more delicious than a steaming bowl of porridge on a cold winter's morning. This recipe, containing iron, essential fatty acids and soluble fibre, is an excellent breakfast for all the family.

**MAKES 1 SERVING**

½ cup of porridge oats
filtered water
1 dessertspoon sunflower seeds and linseeds (flaxseeds), ground
a little formula or breast milk
a drizzle of molasses

Put the oats in a pan with filtered water to cover, and simmer for 5–10 minutes until thickened and cooked through. Place them in a bowl and sprinkle with the ground seeds. (A coffee grinder is a marvellous implement for grinding seeds.)

Surround the porridge with some formula or breast milk and drizzle with a tiny bit of molasses.

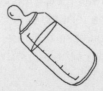

# Baby Muesli

This recipe is rich in essential fatty acids which are particularly important for brain development. These fatty acids are also anti-inflammatory and are therefore a useful aid in the management of inflammatory conditions like asthma and eczema.

**MAKES 1 SERVING**

1 heaped tablespoon porridge oats
2 tablespoons filtered water
1 small ripe banana
½ teaspoon tahini
1 teaspoon flaxseed oil
2 tablespoons breast milk or formula, rice milk or oat milk

Put the oats in a cereal bow, cover with filtered water, and soak overnight. This makes the oats more digestible.

In the morning add all the other ingredients and mash or purée to desired consistency.

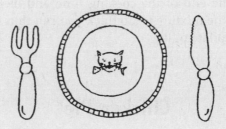

# Lentil Purée*

This lentil purée can be given to a baby from six months onwards. To make it more of a meal for a nine-month-old, you can mix it with some rice, or corn or buckwheat pasta. It also makes a delicious soup for all the family if you replace the water with vegetable stock and double or treble the recipe.

**MAKES 2 PORTIONS TO SERVE WITH PASTA**

1 small onion, peeled and finely chopped
1 small carrot, peeled and finely chopped
1 small stick of celery, trimmed and finely chopped
1 garlic clove, peeled and crushed (optional)
1 teaspoon extra-virgin olive oil
2 tablespoons red lentils
200 ml (7 fl oz) filtered water
1 teaspoon chopped parsley or coriander

Sauté the onion, carrot, celery and garlic (if using), in a little oil for 8–10 minutes. Add the red lentils and the water and cook gently for 15–20 minutes until the lentils are soft. Add the herbs just before the end of the cooking time and blend in a food processor. If the mixture is too thick you can thin it down with a little appropriate milk.

# Chicken Pie*

This is a very quick and easy recipe. You could also use leftover chicken from a roast which would require even less cooking. Use one portion straight away and freeze the extra one. Always take care to reheat cooked chicken until it is piping hot throughout, to avoid the risk of salmonella.

**MAKES 2 INDIVIDUAL PORTIONS**

1 small onion, peeled and chopped
1 teaspoon extra-virgin olive oil
1 small organic chicken breast (boneless and skinless), cubed
1 small carrot, peeled and chopped
1 stick of celery, trimmed and chopped
a handful of frozen peas
300 ml (10 fl oz) filtered water or Chicken Stock (page 96)
1 teaspoon potato flour
1 medium potato
a little appropriate milk
a little unhydrogenated margarine

Sauté the onion in the olive oil until transparent. Add the cubed chicken and sauté for a further 2–3 minutes. Add the rest of the chopped vegetables, the water or stock, and the potato flour (mixed with a little cold water to prevent it getting lumpy). Simmer gently for 25–30 minutes until the chicken is thoroughly cooked and the vegetables tender. You may need to add a little more water or stock if the liquid becomes too thick.

Whilst the chicken is cooking, peel and chop the potato. Put it in a pan, cover with water, bring to the boil and simmer for 20 minutes until soft. Drain and mash with a little appropriate milk and vegetable margarine.

Cover the chicken base with the mashed potato. Cool and serve.

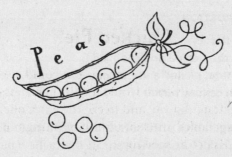

# Carrot, Potato and Tahini

This delicious mixture was an instant hit with my children. You could just as easily bake a potato along with the rest of the family's and mash in some tahini before serving, for an even quicker meal. Tahini (sesame paste) is available from healthfood shops and is an excellent source of calcium, vitamin E and essential fatty acids.

**MAKES 1 PORTION**

1 small carrot
1 small potato
1 teaspoon tahini

Peel and chop the carrot and potato. Steam or boil until cooked and mash or purée to desired consistency. Stir in the tahini before serving.

# Veggies with Cashew Cream

Nut butters are such versatile foods. You can add them to vegetable meals, as in this recipe, or they can be used as spreads. Either make your own (page 181) or, if you prefer, you can buy very good brands of nut butters at healthfood shops.

**MAKES 1 PORTION**

2 broccoli florets
1 small carrot, peeled and chopped
1 small potato, peeled and chopped
1 teaspoon cashew butter

Steam the vegetables until soft. Mash or purée to desired consistency, and just before serving stir in the cashew butter.

# Quick Quinoa*

Quinoa is rich in protein, calcium and iron and is therefore an excellent grain to incorporate in your baby's diet.

**MAKES 2 PORTIONS**

1 small leek, washed well and chopped
1 teaspoon extra-virgin olive oil
1 small courgette, washed and chopped
1 small parsnip, peeled and chopped
1 tablespoon quinoa, washed thoroughly
300 ml (10 fl oz) filtered water

Sauté the leek in the olive oil for 5–10 minutes until soft. Add the rest of the ingredients and simmer for 20–25 minutes until cooked. Mash or purée to desired consistency and serve.

Carrots

# Sweet Potato and Hummus

Yet another favourite! You can now buy excellent ready-made hummus if you are in a hurry.

**MAKES 1 PORTION**

1 small or ½ large sweet potato, peeled and chopped
1 teaspoon Hummus (page 178)

Steam, boil or bake the sweet potato as you would an ordinary potato, mash or purée, and add the hummus before serving.

> **Suggestion**
> This is just as good with ordinary potato.

# Nuts about Pumpkin*

As pumpkins and other squashes tend to be quite large, I have calculated the serving size in ice cubes. This is just a guide and will obviously depend on the size of the squashes used. Adding ground nuts to this recipe boosts the calcium and protein content.

**MAKES ABOUT 36 CUBES**

1 small pumpkin
2 sweet potatoes
1 bunch of well washed watercress, stalks removed
1 teaspoon ground almonds per serving

Wash, peel and chop the pumpkin and sweet potatoes. Steam, with the watercress, until soft and purée in a food processor. Freeze the purée using the ice cube method (page 24).

Defrost 3–6 ice cubes, heat gently, and just before serving add 1 teaspoon ground almonds.

# Buckwheat Pasta and Sauce*

Buckwheat pasta is a good substitute for wheat-based pasta.

**MAKES 2–3 PORTIONS**

a handful of buckwheat pasta
1 tablespoon extra-virgin olive oil
1 small onion, peeled and finely chopped
1 small courgette, washed and chopped
2 tablespoons sugar-free baked beans (e.g. Whole Earth)
2–3 tablespoons filtered water

Cook the buckwheat pasta in a pan of boiling water for 8–10 minutes until soft. Drain. Heat the oil in a pan and sauté the onion and courgette until soft. Add the baked beans, the water and the cooked pasta and simmer gently for 1–2 minutes. Mash or purée to desired consistency.

You could easily make this in bulk and freeze it.

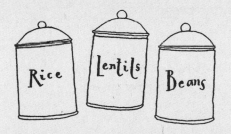

# Sunshine Salad

This recipe is a great introduction to salad and you can use an infinite number of different combinations.

**MAKES 1 PORTION**

¼ of a large or ½ small avocado
1 tablespoon tofu
1 tablespoon canned sweetcorn (no sugar, no salt)
1 tablespoon sprouted beans or seeds (found in healthfood shops or sprout your own – pages 38–40)
1 dark lettuce leaf
a little filtered water

Put all the ingredients into a food processor and blend to the desired consistency.

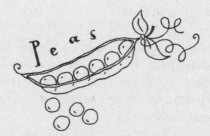

# Avocado, Banana and Tuna

This strange combination is so nutritious and quick to prepare. Older babies will love it.

**MAKES 1 PORTION**

½ avocado
1 small banana
1 tablespoon tinned tuna in water or oil (not brine)

Blend or mash all the ingredients together and serve immediately.

# Vegetarian Iron Booster

This instant iron cocktail can be spread on rice cakes or mixed with grains. Adding a few vitamin C drops will enhance the iron absorption (see Resources for suppliers).

**MAKES 8–10 CUBES**

a handful of spring greens, well cooked and drained
a handful of raisins
1 teaspoon molasses
a little filtered water or cooking water (if necessary)

Blend together the spring greens, raisins and molasses, and serve.

# Salmon Surprise*

Salmon is an excellent introduction to oily fish, being rich in omega 3 essential fatty acids.

**MAKES 3–4 PORTIONS**

1 boneless and skinless salmon fillet
1 small onion
1 teaspoon extra-virgin olive oil
1 small tin sweetcorn (no sugar, no salt)
a handful of frozen peas
1 large potato, peeled and diced
150 ml (5 fl oz) filtered water (with a pinch of low-salt vegetable stock powder added)
1 tablespoon chopped parsley

Bake or steam the salmon fillet for 20–25 minutes (depending on size) until cooked.

Meanwhile, sauté the onion in the olive oil until transparent, add the sweetcorn, peas, diced potato, water and parsley and simmer for 20 minutes until all the vegetables are soft. Add the flaked salmon fillet and simmer for 1–2 more minutes. Mash or purée to desired consistency.

Serve one portion and freeze the remainder.

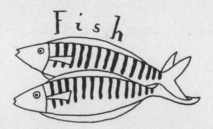

# Iron Booster*

Not many mothers like preparing liver, which is a shame since it is the best dietary source of iron available. If you are a little squeamish, this is an excellent recipe to get you started. But, due to its high vitamin A content, don't give liver to your baby more often than once a fortnight.

**MAKES ABOUT 8 CUBES**

1 organic chicken liver
½ small onion, peeled
1 tablespoon extra-virgin olive oil
3 tablespoons apple juice
1 tablespoon sun-dried raisins or 1 ice cube portion of Dried
  Apricot Purée (page 90)

Remove any sinewy bits from the liver and chop it into small pieces. Finely chop the onion. Then sauté the onion and the liver in the olive oil for 5–10 minutes until cooked. Add the apple juice and the raisins or Dried Apricot Purée ice cube and cook for a further 3–5 minutes. Blend to a fine purée and serve on rice cakes, or add it to a vegetable purée.

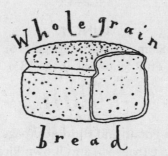

# Sample menus for nine to twelve months

### BREAKFAST
Breast milk or bottle
Oat Porridge (page 106)  Banana pieces

### LUNCH
Slice of roast chicken, mashed potato and broccoli
(e.g. Sunday lunch, mashed or puréed)
Mixture of Apple Purée (page 87) and Date Purée (page 90)
Water

### TEA
Buckwheat Pasta and Sauce (page 113)
Pear Purée (page 91)
Water

### BEDTIME
Breast or bottle

---

### BREAKFAST
Breast or bottle
Baby Muesli (page 107)
Pear pieces

### LUNCH
Salmon Surprise (page 116)
Fruit Smoothie (page 185)
Water

### TEA
Sweet Potato and Hummus (page 112)
Dried Apricot Purée (page 90) and Brown Rice Purée (page 89)
Water

### BEDTIME
Breast or bottle

---

### BREAKFAST
Breast or bottle
Wheat-free baby cereal
Mango slices

### LUNCH
Vegetable Purée (pages 86–89) and Iron Booster (page 117)
Banana and Kiwi Fruit Purée (page 92)
Water

### TEA
Sunshine Salad (page 114)
Baked Apple with Molasses (page 188)
Water

### BEDTIME
Breast or bottle

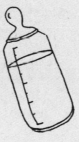

# 5.

# One Year and Older

From the age of one your toddler will enjoy
feeding himself (with your help). Always sit
down and eat with your children, and try to
avoid preparing something different for
yourself. In this chapter you will find recipes
for meat-eaters, vegetarians and vegans,
and there is also a large selection of dairy-free,
wheat-free and gluten-free recipes.

B Y THE AGE OF ONE your toddler will essentially be eating the same as everyone else in the family. You can now introduce whole cow's milk, goat's milk or fortified soya milk instead of formula or breast milk. You can also introduce wheat-based products like bread, pasta and flour, but try to keep them down to one meal a day. This will encourage you to give your toddler plenty of variety in his diet. Remember to be cautious with any other new foods that can produce an allergic reaction (like eggs) and give just a little for the first try.

From the age of one your toddler will enjoy feeding himself (with your help). Please don't be alarmed if he suddenly becomes fiercely independent and insists on feeding himself entirely. This happens more often than not and you just need to be prepared for a little more mess. Switching to mainly finger food meals until he has got the hang of cutlery can be a real relief! He will also be drinking capably from a feeder cup at meal-times. Only offer water or milk at mealtimes. It is unnecessary to introduce diluted fruit juices at this age. Between 14 and 18 months most toddlers can progress from high chair to booster seat and eat at the table with the rest of the family.

You may find that after the age of one your toddler's appetite becomes less consistent. Most mothers worry about how much their child is eating. This is quite natural. However, if your toddler's eating habits turn a little erratic, view his diet in terms of what he eats in a week rather than a day. I know that some days my children seem to eat very little, and other days they eat the same quantity as me. There's usually no need to get anxious. Children do eat when they are hungry. But if they are coming down with an illness, are cross, tired or even just having too much fun playing, food will take second place on their list of priorities. By being relaxed about it, you will avoid any potential food battles.

Always sit down and eat with your children, and try to avoid preparing something different for yourself. Your toddler will inevitably find the food on your plate more interesting than the food on his! Children do what we do, not what we say, however much we sometimes wish they wouldn't! For this reason, you will find that the recipes in this section, unless stated otherwise, cater for the average family – two adults and two children.

## The dairy debate

In the West, cow's milk, and other products made from it (like butter, cheese and yogurt) are assumed to be an essential part of a child's diet, providing a good source of protein, fat and carbohydrate and a vital source of calcium. However, with the huge increase in childhood complaints like asthma, eczema, ear infections and most recently, childhood diabetes, some doctors and health professionals are questioning the role that dairy products play in our children's diet. The government now recommends that whole cow's milk is not introduced as a drink before the age of one. I believe that no child should be exposed to any dairy products at all before the age of one. Dairy products are difficult to digest, highly mucus-forming and inflammatory by nature.

It's really very easy to maintain adequate calcium levels whilst avoiding dairy products. And, once past the age of one, it is quite safe to avoid dairy products as long as you are extremely vigilant and make sure your child has a varied diet containing lots of calcium-rich foods. As you can see from the list below, there are many sources of calcium other than dairy products. The advantage of using some plant-based sources is that these foods generally contain good levels of magnesium which helps the body absorb the calcium.

## Calcium found in everyday foods

| Food | Amount (g)* | Calcium (mg)* |
|---|---|---|
| Cow's milk | 100 | 115 |
| Cheddar cheese | 100 | 720 |
| Fromage frais | 100 | 86 |
| Kale | 100 | 150 |
| Watercress (raw) | 100 | 170 |
| Spinach (boiled) | 100 | 160 |
| Spring greens (raw) | 100 | 210 |
| Sesame seeds | 100 | 670 |
| Tahini paste | 100 | 680 |
| Almonds | 100 | 240 |
| Brazil nuts | 100 | 170 |
| Calcium-enriched soya milk | 100 (ml) | 140 |
| Tofu (precipitated with calcium) | 100 | 150 |
| Sardines (canned in oil) | 100 | 550 |
| Pilchards (canned in tomato sauce) | 100 | 300 |
| Molasses | 1 tablespoon | 140 |

*100 g is equivalent to 3.5 oz, 100 ml is equivalent to 3.5 fl oz.

**The recommended nutrient intake of calcium for a 1–3 year old is 350 mg, and for a 4–6 year old is 450 mg.

Adapted from McCance and Widdowson's *The Composition of Foods* (5th edition) and manufacturer's labels.

## Dairy alternatives to use for drinking and cooking

**Soya milk:** Use calcium-enriched. Soya milk slightly sweetened with apple juice seems to be the favourite and is good on cereals and sweeter dishes. The unsweetened variety is recommended for savoury cooking.

**Rice milk:** Delicious as a drink or on cereals. Too thin to cook with.

**Oat milk:** Very thick, oaty drink. Good on cereals and useful in baking.

**Almond milk:** (See recipes). Useful as a drink, milkshake or cream alternative.

**Coconut milk:** Very rich and needs to be diluted 1:3 with water. It makes a good alternative to cream and is delicious in sauces or puddings.

**Unhydrogenated margarines:** Good for spreading and several varieties are now available for cooking.

**Soya yogurts:** Live natural yogurt available as well as fruit varieties.

**Soya cheese:** Hard cheeses as well as cream cheeses available.

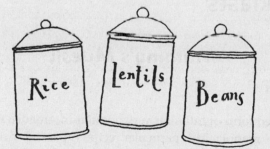

## Recipes one year and older

This section contains the bulk of the recipes, all designed to serve a family of two adults and two children. If you are catering for more or less, the recipes can easily be adapted by halving or doubling. Many of them, as indicated, can be frozen or kept for a few days in the fridge.

There are dishes for meat-eaters, vegetarians and vegans, and there is also a large selection of dairy-free, wheat-free and gluten-free recipes, as indicated by the symbols below.

## Key

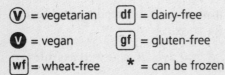

Ⓥ = vegetarian    df = dairy-free

🅥 = vegan    gf = gluten-free

wf = wheat-free    * = can be frozen

# Breakfasts

## Mummy's Muesli

Ⓥ 🅥 df

This baked form of muesli is very popular in America where it is known as granola. This particular recipe is packed with protein, essential fats, B vitamins and trace minerals. A perfect high-energy breakfast for active youngsters, it does not last very long in our house! Keep it in the fridge once made to protect the essential fatty acids in the nuts and seeds. For this recipe, like many others, please don't worry about measurements, a few more or less oats will make no difference.

**MAKES 8 CUPS OF MUESLI**

3 cups of oats
1 cup of wheatgerm
¼ cup of sesame seeds
¼ cup of linseeds
¼ cup of sunflower seeds
4 tablespoons ground almonds
1 tablespoon barley malt (dissolved in a little warm water, as it is very sticky otherwise)
1 tablespoon crude blackstrap molasses (dissolved in a little warm water as above)
¼ cup extra-virgin olive oil or walnut oil
1 teaspoon natural vanilla extract
1 teaspoon ground cinnamon
2 cups of raisins
½ cup of dessicated coconut

Preheat the oven to 180°C/350°F/Gas Mark 4.

Mix the oats, wheatgerm, seeds and almonds in a large bowl. Combine the barley malt, molasses, oil, vanilla and cinnamon in a separate bowl. Mix the wet ingredients with the dry, stirring well until all the ingredients are well coated with the oil.

Spread the mixture out on two baking trays. Bake for 20 minutes or until golden-brown, stirring after 10 minutes.

Add the raisins and coconut and allow to cool. Once cooled, place in an airtight jar or tin in the fridge. Serve topped with whole milk, goat's milk, soya milk, rice milk, live yogurt or fresh juice.

## Best of the bought breakfast cereals

These are mainly available in healthfood shops and are free from additives, added sugar and salt:

Porridge oats, millet flakes, puffed rice cereal, Kashi multigrain cereal, cornflakes without added sugar, baby muesli (e.g. Familia), sugar-free muesli (e.g. Whole Earth).

# Raw Muesli

(V) wf df

This recipe is a variation on the famous muesli developed by Dr Max Bircher-Benner for the benefit of patients at his clinic in Zurich. It is delicious and adored by children and adults alike. If you wish to make this dairy-free, use soya milk, almond milk, diluted coconut milk or rice milk instead of whole milk.

8 heaped tablespoons oat flakes
filtered water
2 small handfuls of sun-dried raisins
2 apples, peeled and grated
2 small bananas, mashed
1 tablespoon cold-pressed honey or blackstrap molasses
8 tablespoons whole milk, soya milk or rice milk
2 tablespoons ground almonds, or chopped nuts or sunflower
    seeds (optional)
a pinch of ground cinnamon or ginger (optional)

Cover the oats with filtered water and soak overnight to help break the starches down into sugars, along with the raisins. In the morning, the mixture should be really gooey, not water-logged!

Combine the soaked mixture with the fruit. Drizzle with honey or molasses. Add a little milk. Sprinkle with nuts or seeds, and spices if you wish.

There are endless variations to this recipe. You can use any fruit in place of the banana: grated pear, fresh berries, peaches or even dried fruit.

# Tofu Scramble

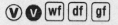

This is a very quick high-protein breakfast which is a good alternative to egg. Serve it immediately with wholewheat toast, gluten-free toast, fresh soda bread, rice cakes, oat cakes or rye crackers.

> 1 onion, peeled and finely chopped
> 1 tablespoon extra-virgin olive oil
> a pinch of turmeric
> 100 g (4 oz) block of firm tofu, mashed

In a frying pan lightly fry the onion in the olive oil until transparent. Sprinkle over the turmeric and add the mashed tofu. Lightly fry, stirring well for a couple of minutes.

---

**Suggestion**

You could also do this recipe without onion. Add a pinch of low-salt Marigold Swiss vegetable bouillon powder for flavour.

---

# Meal-in-One Soups

## Lentil Soup*

(V) (V) wf df gf

This soup is very warm and comforting on a cold winter's day, and lentils are a great source of iron. Serve it with fresh soda bread or wholewheat rolls for a light lunch.

1 onion, peeled and chopped
1 garlic clove, peeled and chopped
1 tablespoon extra-virgin olive oil
1 carrot, peeled and chopped
2 sticks of celery, finely chopped
100 g (4 oz) red lentils
600 ml (1 pint) low-salt Marigold Swiss vegetable bouillon
a handful of chopped parsley or coriander

Sauté the onion and garlic in the olive oil until the onion is transparent. Add the vegetables, lentils and bouillon. Cover, bring to the boil and gently simmer for 20–25 minutes until the vegetables are tender and the lentils have turned a pale orange.

Add the chopped parsley or coriander and blend in a food processor until smooth and creamy. You may want to add more stock or water if it is too thick.

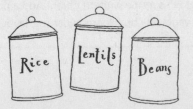

# Nutty Leek, Potato and Parsnip Soup*

(V) (V) [wf] [df] [gf]

This is a variation on traditional leek and potato soup. The parsnip adds a natural sweetness which children love. And the addition of a nut or seed butter makes the soup more of a meal and boosts its nutritional content.

2 small leeks, washed and sliced
2 tablespoons olive oil
2 large potatoes, peeled and chopped
1 large parsnip, peeled and chopped
600 ml (1 pint) low-salt Marigold Swiss vegetable bouillon
cashew nut butter or tahini
croûtons
chopped parsley

Sauté the leeks in the oil for 2–3 minutes. Add the potatoes and parsnips and cover with stock. Simmer for half an hour until soft. When cooked, liquidise in a food processor to a nice thick consistency. Thin it down a little with some water or extra stock if you want to. I find that if it isn't really thick it runs off the children's spoons and makes a huge mess!

Just before serving, stir a teaspoon of cashew nut butter or tahini into each bowl and sprinkle with croûtons and chopped parsley.

## Croûton ideas

Diced wholewheat toast, small chunks of rice cake, or Oatcake Fingers or Animals (page 183). Children love to help themselves at mealtimes and this is a good way of introducing involvement.

# Roasted Red Pepper and Squash Soup*

Ⓥ Ⓥ ⟨wf⟩ ⟨df⟩ ⟨gf⟩

Children love the natural sweetness of this soup. It is rich in beta-carotene (which is important for the healing process) and the roasted red peppers give it a wonderful flavour. It also freezes well.

  1 red pepper, in half, deseeded and destalked
  2 tablespoons extra-virgin olive oil
  1 large onion, peeled and chopped
  1 carrot, peeled and chopped
  1 small squash (can be butternut, kaboucha or a small pumpkin),
    peeled and chopped
  600 ml (1 pint) low-salt Marigold Swiss vegetable bouillon (you
    may need to add more, depending on the size of your
    vegetables)
  chopped parsley

Preheat the oven to 180°C/350°F/Gas Mark 4. Brush the two pieces of red pepper with 1 tablespoon of the olive oil and place in the oven on a baking sheet to roast for 20–30 minutes.

Meanwhile, chop the onion and sauté in 1 tablespoon of the olive oil until transparent. Add the carrot, squash and stock and simmer for 25 minutes until all the vegetables are soft. Add more stock if necessary.

When the pepper halves are cooked, take their skins off, chop the flesh, and add it to the soup. Liquidise the soup in a food processor and serve with some fresh parsley sprinkled over the top.

# Immune-boosting Soup

Ⓥ Ⓥ wf df

This is an ideal soup when your children are below par. The hummus adds creaminess and colour as well as iron, calcium and protein.

1 onion, peeled and chopped
1 clove of garlic, peeled and crushed
1 tablespoon extra-virgin olive oil
1 slice of ginger, peeled and chopped
1 carrot, peeled and chopped
1 stick of celery, chopped
1 potato, peeled and cubed
a handful of pot barley
600–850 ml (1–1½ pints) low-salt Marigold Swiss vegetable
  bouillon
a head of broccoli, broken into florets
a handful of chopped parsley
1 heaped tablespoon hummus (optional)

Sauté the onion and garlic in the olive oil until transparent. Add all the other ingredients except the broccoli, parsley and hummus, and stir well. Cover and simmer for 40 minutes.

Add the broccoli and cook for a further 5–10 minutes.

Just before serving, sprinkle over the parsley and stir in the hummus.

# Minestrone with Pesto

(V) [wf] [df] [gf]

This is quite a labour-intensive recipe, but delicious all the same. It is even more delicious with fresh walnut pesto. Use rice pasta shells or corn pasta shells if you're trying to avoid wheat.

1 tablespoon extra-virgin olive oil
1 onion, peeled and chopped
2 garlic cloves, peeled and crushed
1 tablespoon fresh rosemary
1 × 425 g (15 oz) can chickpeas (no sugar, no salt)
850 ml (1½ pints) low-salt Marigold Swiss vegetable bouillon
4 ripe tomatoes skinned and chopped
1 courgette, diced
50 g (2 oz) shelled fresh peas (or frozen)
50 g (2 oz) French beans
50 g (2 oz) shelled broad beans
50 g (2 oz) small wheat, rice or corn pasta shells
2 tablespoons chopped fresh parsley
green pesto or fresh Walnut Pesto (page 137)

Heat the oil in a large pan, add the onion, garlic and rosemary, and sauté gently for 5 minutes until softened and transparent. Add the chickpeas, the stock, and the tomatoes and bring to the boil. Cover and simmer for 30 minutes.

Add the courgette, peas and beans to the soup. Return to the boil and simmer for a further 10 minutes. Add the pasta and parsley and cook for a further 6–8 minutes until the pasta is cooked. Season if necessary.

Just before serving, add a teaspoon of green pesto or Walnut Pesto to each bowl and stir in.

# Courgette Soup*

Ⓥ Ⓥ wf df gf

This recipe looks so ordinary but it comes out as thick and creamy as if you had added a pint of cream. You can freeze it but it tends to turn rather watery so I'd advise against it. Serve with chunky croûtons. Max (my son) likes to spread mini rice cakes with peanut butter and then watch them floating on the top!

1 large or 2 medium onions, peeled and chopped
1 tablespoon extra-virgin olive oil
675 g (1½ lb) courgettes, diced
600 ml (1 pint) low-salt Marigold Swiss vegetable bouillon

Sauté the onion in the oil until transparent. Then add the courgettes and the stock. Simmer for half an hour and liquidise.

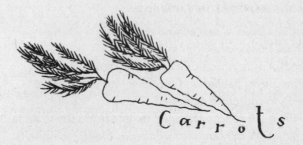

Carrots

# Pasta Sauces

## Quick and Easy Pasta Sauce*

(V) (V) [wf] [df] [gf]

This recipe has been a particular favourite with both my children. It is also a very good way to ensure that plenty of vegetables get eaten! The easiest way to use it is to freeze individual portions for an instant meal. Ring the changes with the pasta you serve to ensure that you are not giving your child too much wheat. There are plenty of wheat-free varieties available now from supermarkets and healthfood shops, including corn pasta, rice and vegetable pasta, buckwheat (soba) pasta and spinach and barley pasta.

**MAKES ABOUT 8–10 FREEZER PORTIONS
(2–3 TABLESPOONS IN EACH POT)**

2 medium onions, peeled and chopped
2 tablespoons extra-virgin olive oil
a handful of mushrooms, wiped and chopped
1 large carrot, peeled and chopped into small pieces
1 medium courgette, chopped
1 × 400 g (14 oz) can chopped tomatoes (no sugar, no salt)
1 × 425 g (15 oz) can flageolot beans (no sugar, no salt)
1 tablespoon chopped fresh parsley

Fry the onions in the oil until transparent. Add the mushrooms and cook for 2–3 minutes. Add the carrot and courgette and coat with oil. Pour in the chopped tomatoes and beans and simmer until the vegetables are soft. Toss in the parsley and whizz up in a food processor until smooth.

> **Suggestions**
>
> You can use this recipe as a base for many other pasta sauces. Instead of the flageolet beans, you could use some cooked chicken, cooked lamb or cooked chicken liver, and purée in the food processor as above.

# Walnut Pesto*

Ⓥ wf gf

Walnuts are a good source of omega 3 essential fatty acids which are important not only for your child's immune system, but also his hair, skin and brain function. This pesto keeps for up to a week in the fridge. Serve it with fresh spinach tagliatelle.

A really delicious alternative is to use fresh rocket instead of the basil. You will need about 100 g (4 oz) rocket. Adults will love it too.

    25 g (1 oz) or ¼ cup walnuts
    25 g (1 oz) or ¼ cup grated parmesan
    2 × 50 g (2 oz) supermarket packets of fresh basil
    1–2 garlic cloves (depending on your family's preference)
    50 ml (2 fl oz) or ¼ cup extra-virgin olive oil

Grind the walnuts finely in a food processor. Add the rest of the ingredients and mix until you have a smooth, slightly grainy paste. You may want to add more olive oil if it is too thick. I usually just drizzle the oil through the top of the food processor until the pesto reaches the consistency I like.

## Other pasta sauce ideas

Vegetable Rich Mince (page 166)
Vegetarian Spaghetti Bolognese (page 146)
Salmon Pesto Spaghetti (page 174)
Roasted vegetables and grated parmesan (see Mediterranean
   Ratatouille Bake, page 152)
Instant Fishy Pasta Sauce (page 174)
Bean Stew (page 142)

# Main Meals (Vegetarian)

## Sunshine Tofu Risotto

(V) (V) [wf] [df] [gf]

Even the very young will enjoy this recipe, as the vegetables and
rice become very soft, and it is so colourful. Serve with a large
salad.

   1 block of firm tofu
   1 onion, peeled and chopped
   1 clove garlic, peeled and crushed
   2 tablespoons extra-virgin olive oil
   225 g (8 oz) or 1 cup easy-cook brown rice
   1 × 200 g (7 oz) tin sweetcorn (no sugar, no salt)
   3 tablespoons frozen or fresh peas
   5 mushrooms, wiped and chopped
   1 small courgette, diced
   1 small red pepper, deseeded and diced
   900 ml (1½ pints) low-salt Marigold Swiss vegetable bouillon
   a handful of fresh coriander, basil or parsley

Drain the tofu and squeeze any excess moisture out of it. Chop the tofu into small cubes. Fry the onion and garlic in the oil until transparent. Add the tofu and cook for a further 3 minutes.

Add the rice and coat with oil. Toss in the vegetables and add the stock. Cook gently until all the stock has been absorbed and the rice is cooked. Once cooked, stir in the herbs and serve.

> **Suggestion**
> You can replace the tofu with leftover chicken to make a Chicken Risotto.

# Home-made Chips

Ⓥ Ⓥ wf df gf

These healthy oven chips are so quick to prepare and free from salt and heat-damaged oils. Served with baked beans and some salad, they make a quick and nutritious tea for toddlers.

2 large potatoes
2 sweet potatoes
extra-virgin olive oil (for brushing)
a pinch of dried oregano

Preheat the oven to 190°C/375°F/Gas Mark 5. Keeping the skins on (if organic), chop the potatoes into thick chip shapes. Brush on both sides with the oil and sprinkle with the oregano.

Bake in the oven for 40–50 minutes (longer if you are doing a larger quantity), turning once or twice to prevent sticking, until the chips are golden-brown and soft in the middle.

# Vegetable Casserole*

(V) (v) [wf] [df] [gf]

Children love the sweetness of this casserole and it is wonderfully warming on a cold winter's day, served with brown rice, buckwheat, millet or quinoa.

1 onion, peeled and chopped
1 tablespoon extra-virgin olive oil
450 g (1 lb) mixed root vegetables (e.g. potatoes, carrots, sweet potato, swede, parsnip, turnip, celery or whatever root vegetables you have in the fridge), peeled and chopped
600 ml (1 pint) low-salt Marigold Swiss vegetable bouillon
1 tablespoon potato flour
1 × 425 g (15 oz) tin of mixed beans (no salt, no sugar)

Fry the onion in the oil until transparent. Add the chopped root vegetables and cover with the stock. Mix the potato flour with a little cold water to prevent lumps and pour into the casserole. Add the beans and bake in the oven at 160°C/325°F/Gas Mark 3 for 2 hours.

---

### Suggestion

This also makes a delicious soup. Just purée the mixture in the food processor if your children do not like the look of beans!

# Herby Millet

(V) wf df gf

This is a dairy- and wheat-free recipe which is delicious served with a vegetable stew or ratatouille. Millet is such an alkaline grain, kind to the digestive system and rich in potassium, iron, calcium and the B vitamins. I love to use fresh green herbs wherever possible in recipes as they introduce the children to a variety of flavours and are rich in iron and calcium.

175 g (6 oz) millet
600 ml (1 pint) low-salt Marigold Swiss vegetable bouillon
1 large onion, peeled and chopped
2 tablespoons extra-virgin olive oil
1 organic egg (optional)
a handful of chopped coriander or parsley

Gently cook the millet in the stock for 25 minutes. Whilst the millet is cooking, soften the onion in the oil. Once the millet has absorbed all the stock (if it needs more, just add a little water), add the onion, the beaten egg (if using) and the herbs. Stir for a couple of minutes to cook the egg and serve immediately.

If you leave out the egg, you can bake the millet in the oven for 10–15 minutes, at 190°C/375°F/Gas Mark 5, before serving to give it a crusty top.

Carrots

# Bean Stew*

Ⓥ Ⓥ wf gf

This recipe takes no time at all to throw together. It can be served with brown rice, millet, buckwheat or quinoa, or alternatively, you can use it as a pasta topping.

    1 tablespoon extra-virgin olive oil
    1 onion, peeled and chopped
    a handful of mushrooms, wiped and chopped
    1 courgette, chopped
    2 × 400 g (14 oz) cans tinned tomatoes (no sugar, no salt)
    1 × 425 g (15 oz) can mixed pulses (no sugar, no salt)
    chopped parsley

Heat the oil and sauté the onion, mushrooms and courgette for a few minutes until the onion is transparent. Add the tomatoes and the pulses, cook for 20 minutes on a low heat, and serve, garnished with some chopped parsley.

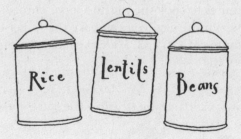

# Nut Roast

(V) (V) [df]

If you have a food processor, this takes no time at all to prepare and is utterly delicious for all the family. This recipe makes 6–8 good slices. Serve with a crunchy salad and sugar-free tomato sauce.

4 small slices wholemeal bread
225 g (8 oz) mixed nuts, finely chopped
a bunch of spring onions, trimmed and washed
1 carrot, finely grated
1 clove garlic, peeled
2 medium tomatoes, skinned
a handful of parsley

Put the slices of wholemeal bread into the food processor and chop to fine breadcrumbs. Pour out into a large bowl. Lightly roast the nuts under the grill for a few minutes and then finely grind them in the food processor. Add them to the breadcrumbs.

Next, chop the spring onion, grated carrot, garlic, tomatoes and parsley in the food processor for a minute until finely chopped. Don't leave it on too long or you will be left with a runny mush!

Add the wet ingredients to the dry and mix well with your hands. Transfer to a non-stick loaf tin, press down well, cover with foil and bake for 1 hour at 190°C/375°F/Gas Mark 5, removing the foil after half an hour to allow the top to brown.

# Lentil Shepherd's Pie

Ⓥ wf df gf

This is an all-time family favourite and so much nicer than it sounds! It freezes well without the mashed potato. And if you substitute tamari soy sauce for the Worcestershire sauce, the recipe is truly vegetarian. (Worcestershire sauce contains anchovy extract.)

100 g (4 oz) green lentils
450 g (1 lb) potatoes
1 large onion, peeled and chopped
1 clove garlic, peeled and crushed
1 tablespoon olive oil
a handful of mushrooms, wiped and chopped
1 × 400 g (14 oz) can chopped tomatoes (no sugar, no salt)
1 tablespoon tomato purée
1 tablespoon Worcestershire sauce or tamari soy sauce
a bunch of parsley, chopped
a little unhydrogenated margarine
soya or nut milk

Put the lentils in a pan, cover with water and simmer for 45 minute until soft. Drain and put to one side.

Meanwhile, peel and chop the potatoes, put them in a pan, with water to cover, and bring to the boil. Set the oven to 190°C/375°F/Gas Mark 5. Sauté the onion and garlic in the olive oil until transparent. Add the mushrooms and cook for a further 2 minutes. Add the tomatoes, tomato purée, Worcestershire sauce or soy sauce, and the cooked lentils. Finally, add half the parsley and cook for a few more minutes.

Take off the heat while you drain and mash the potatoes with a little margarine and soya milk (or non-dairy alternative) ready for the top of the pie. Pour the lentil mixture into an ovenproof dish and place the mashed potato on top.

Bake for 30 minutes until the potato has started to turn a golden-brown. Just before serving, toss the rest of the parsley over the top for added colour.

# Roasted Root Veggies with Dips

Ⓥ Ⓥ wf df gf

Another quick and nutritious tea.

> 1 sweet potato, 1 parsnip, 1 carrot and 2 potatoes
> 2 tablespoons extra-virgin olive oil

Preheat the oven to 190°C/375°F/Gas Mark 5.

Peel (unless they are organic) and chop the vegetables into chunky-size chips. Roll in the olive oil and bake in the oven for 40–50 minutes until cooked.

Serve straightaway with a variety of dips like Hummus (page 178), Guacamole (page 179), Peanut Butter Dip (page 178), and Veg and Nut Paté (page 180). Accompany the roasted veggies with some crudités to dip as well, e.g. celery, cucumber and carrot sticks.

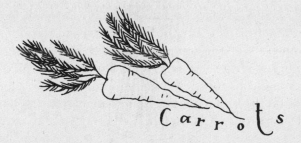

Carrots

# Vegetarian Spaghetti Bolognese*

(V) (V) [df]

This recipe freezes really well for another instant meal. Serve with corn pasta shells or buckwheat spirals.

75 g (3 oz) dried soya mince (TVP)
1 onion, peeled and chopped
1 clove garlic, peeled and crushed
1 tablespoon extra-virgin olive oil
2 tablespoons tomato purée
a handful of mushrooms, wiped and chopped
1 carrot, peeled and chopped
1 × 400 g (14 oz) can tinned tomatoes
2 teaspoons natural gravy browning, diluted in a little cold water
a handful of fresh parsley, chopped

Rehydrate the mince by soaking it in boiling water for 1 minute. Drain.

Sauté the onion and garlic in the oil until transparent. Add the rest of the ingredients, simmer for 20–25 minutes, and serve.

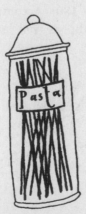

> **Suggestion**
> Pop some mashed potato (made with soya milk) on the top and you
> have a vegan shepherd's pie.

# Wholemeal Quiche

(V) [df]

This is a really quick dish if you buy wholemeal pastry cases for
your storecupboard. They are available from healthfood shops.

> 1 tablespoon extra-virgin olive oil
> a mixture of vegetables (chopped onions, broccoli florets, grated
> carrot, grated swede, sweetcorn, chopped peppers, chopped
> mushrooms, etc.)
> 1 large wholemeal pastry flan case
> 2 tablespoons cooked adzuki beans or chickpeas
> 3 organic eggs
> a splash of milk or soya milk

Heat the oil, sauté the onion, then add the rest of the vegetables
and sauté for about 5 minutes until soft. Pour into the pastry
case and toss the beans or chickpeas over the top. Beat the
eggs and the milk together and pour over to cover the vegetable
mixture.

Bake in the oven for 30 minutes at 180°C/350°F/Gas Mark 4.

> **Suggestion**
> You can easily replace the beans with some tinned tuna or grated
> cheese.

# Millet Burgers

(V) [wf]

Millet makes an excellent alternative to breadcrumbs in burgers of all types. This is another wheat-free recipe.

  1 onion, peeled and finely chopped
  100 g (4 oz) organic Cheddar cheese, grated
  175 g (6 oz) millet grain
  ¼ teaspoon English mustard powder
  1 tablespoon chopped parsley
  1 organic egg, beaten

Mix the ingredients together, either by hand or in the food processor. Form into burger shapes. If they are a little mushy, chill in the fridge for 1 hour before cooking.

  Grill under a medium grill for 10 minutes each side. Alternatively, bake in the oven for 15–25 minutes at 190°C/375°F/Gas Mark 5.

# Tofu Fingers

(V) [df]

These are very easy to prepare and free from any artificial flavours, colours or preservatives.

  1–2 × 225 g (8 oz) blocks firm tofu
  4 tablespoons plain flour, seasoned with mixed dried herbs
  2 organic eggs, beaten with a splash of soy sauce
  1–2 slices wholemeal bread, made into breadcrumbs
  extra-virgin olive oil or butter (for frying)

Slice the tofu into finger shapes. Prepare three shallow dishes: one with flour, one with beaten egg and one with the breadcrumbs. Roll the tofu fingers in the flour first, then the egg, and finally in the breadcrumbs until well coated.

Fry gently in a little olive oil or butter, turning occasionally, for 10–15 minutes.

# Potato Cakes

(V) (V) wf df

This is a great tea-time dish for children. You can make it from scratch but it's even quicker if you have some leftover mashed potato in the fridge.

> 450 g (1 lb) potatoes, mashed with a knob of butter and a little
>   milk or dairy-free alternatives
> 100 g (4 oz) cashew nuts, ground
> 2 tablespoons chopped parsley
> 1 carrot, peeled and finely grated
> 1 small onion, peeled and finely chopped
> butter or extra-virgin olive oil (for frying)

Cook the potatoes and mash with the butter and milk to get a firm consistency. Stir in the remaining ingredients and form into small burger shapes. Pop in the fridge before cooking if they need firming up.

Fry for 5 minutes on each side or grill for a little longer.

# Chinese Stir-fry with Tofu (or Chicken)

(V) (V) wf df gf

This is a delicious recipe which older children love eating with chopsticks. Even my three- and four-year-old like to try them out. If you have a child who does not like vegetables that much, it is a wonderful distraction. I often make this dish when we have children to tea, as it can be great fun! Serve it with brown rice, couscous (wheat-based), millet or amaranth.

1 × 225 g (8 oz) block firm tofu, drained and marinated
2 tablespoons cold-pressed runny honey
2 tablespoons tamari soy sauce (wheat-free)
2 garlic cloves, peeled and crushed
some grated ginger
2 tablespoons olive oil
1 onion, peeled and sliced
1 red pepper, deseeded and sliced
1 yellow pepper, deseeded and sliced
a few mushrooms, sliced
a large handful of beansprouts
a stick of celery, chopped
1 carrot, peeled and sliced

First cut the already drained tofu into cubes. Put 1 tablespoon honey, 1 tablespoon soy sauce, 1 crushed garlic clove and some grated ginger into a bowl and stir the tofu into the mixture until well coated. Leave to marinate for a couple of hours before cooking.

Heat the oil in a wok and add the onion, garlic and tofu and stir for 1 minute. Add the rest of the vegetables and stir for a couple of minutes. Add the remaining honey and soy sauce and stir-fry for another 2 minutes.

## Quick tip

If you are in a hurry, you can buy ready-marinated tofu in the super-market. It is usually with the cheese in the refrigerated section.

## Suggestion

Use a diced chicken breast instead of the tofu but stir-fry the chicken for a little longer to ensure thorough cooking.

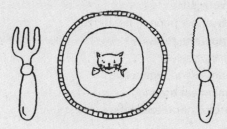

# Mediterranean Ratatouille Bake

Ⓥ

This is such a colourful dish and very rich in antioxidant nutrients. With the addition of the garlic, it is a really good 'keep the bugs at bay' recipe. It takes a little while to prepare as there is quite a lot of chopping to do but the taste is worth every minute. It's also good for entertaining because you can make the ratatouille in advance and put the topping on at the last minute.

1 small aubergine
2 large onions, peeled
1 medium courgette
1 red and 1 yellow pepper, deseeded
6 smallish ripe tomatoes
2 cloves garlic, peeled
3 tablespoons extra-virgin olive oil
3 slices wholemeal bread
a large handful of grated cheese

Preheat the oven to 190°C/375°F/Gas Mark 5.

Chop all the vegetables into cubes. Crush the garlic into the baking tray, add the oil and the vegetables and toss them until all coated with the oil (add a little more if necessary). Bake, uncovered, for 45 minutes until soft. (The smell is quite wonderful!)

Put into an ovenproof dish. Mix the breadcrumbs together with the grated cheese and spread over the top of the vegetable mixture. Bake in the oven for 15 minutes or until crispy on the top.

# Beany Bake

Ⓥ

This is such a quick storecupboard recipe and is always an instant hit – even with the anti-bean brigade. Serve with a crispy salad.

1 × 425 g (15 oz) tin of baked beans (no sugar)
1 × 200 g (7 oz) tin of sweetcorn (no sugar, no salt)
4 slices wholemeal bread, made into breadcrumbs
100 g (4 oz) organic Cheddar cheese, grated

Put the beans and the sweetcorn into an ovenproof dish. Cover with the breadcrumbs and the cheese and bake in the oven for 20 minutes at 190°C/375°F/Gas Mark 5.

> **Suggestion**
> For a wheat-free variation, slice cooked potatoes on top. Some children prefer this – mine certainly do!

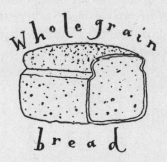

# Vegetable Frittata

(V)

This is a really quick and easy Saturday lunch for all the family. For a family of four, I would use six eggs. Serve the frittata chopped into wedges with a salad and some fresh diluted orange juice, rich in vitamin C, to ensure good iron absorption from the egg.

1 small onion, peeled and chopped
1 tablespoon extra-virgin olive oil
1 small carrot, peeled and grated
a handful of mini broccoli florets or chopped French beans
½ courgette, grated
2 tablespoons tinned sweetcorn (no sugar, no salt)
6 organic eggs
a splash of whole milk or soya milk
chopped parsley, coriander or basil

In a deep frying pan, gently sauté the onion in the olive oil. Add the rest of the vegetables and allow them to sweat for a few minutes. Beat the eggs with a little milk and pour over the vegetables. Swirl the egg around the pan so that the runny egg in the middle reaches an outside edge. Sprinkle the fresh herbs over the top. Cover and cook gently for about 15 minutes until set. If you are brave you can try to turn it over!

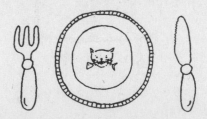

# Boston Baked Beans*

Ⓥ Ⓥ df

It might sound like a waste of time to make your own baked beans but if you have a large, heavy casserole dish you can make these in bulk and pop small portions in the deep freeze. This recipe makes 15–20 children's portions. They smell so wonderful when they're cooking and my children love them. The bonus is that they are low in sugar, and high in fibre, calcium and iron. This recipe works just as well if halved.

1 × 450 g (1 lb) packet dried haricot beans (soaked overnight) or
    4 × 425 g (15 oz) tins haricot beans (no sugar, no salt)
3 medium onions, peeled and finely chopped
4 cloves garlic, peeled and crushed
3 tablespoons extra-virgin olive oil
2 level teaspoons ground paprika
600 ml (1 pint) filtered water
2 tablespoons molasses
2 heaped tablespoons organic, sugar-free tomato ketchup
3 tablespoons tomato purée

If using dried, pre-soaked beans, drain and rinse them, put them in a pan, cover with water and simmer for an hour until cooked. Drain and leave on one side until required.

On top of the stove, fry the onions and garlic in the oil in a large, heavy casserole dish until lightly browned. Add the paprika and a little filtered water to make a rich sauce. Add the molasses, tomato ketchup and tomato purée and add water, little by little, to make a thickish sauce.

Add the beans and the rest of the water and bake in the oven at 150°C/300°F/Gas Mark 2 for 2 hours until cooked. You may have to add a little more water after an hour's cooking.

# Baked Eggs

Ⓥ df

This is a really quick teatime dish that I loved as a child and still do. Serve with whole-grain toast and raw vegetable sticks. To make it dairy-free use the alternatives suggested.

1 × 400 g (14 oz) tin of sweetcorn (no sugar, no salt)
6 organic eggs
a knob of butter or unhydrogenated margarine
a splash of whole milk or soya milk

Grease 4 ramekin dishes. Divide the sweetcorn between the ramekins, evenly distributed in the bottom, and crack an egg on the top (adults will probably want two eggs). Put a little butter or margarine on top of the eggs and a splash of milk around the sides. Bake for 10–15 minutes at 180°C/350°F/Gas Mark 4.

# Summer Salads

## Salad Dressing

Ⓥ Ⓥ wf df gf

This dressing got my youngest interested in salad. A little goes a long way. (This recipe makes about 10 tablespoons of dressing.)

1 dessertspoon Dijon mustard
1 dessertspoon cold-pressed runny honey
1 small clove of garlic, peeled and crushed
3 tablespoons apple cider vinegar
6 tablespoons extra-virgin olive oil (or flaxseed oil, or sunflower)

Mix together the mustard, honey and garlic to form a smooth paste. Slowly add the cider vinegar, mixing until you get a smooth sauce. Add the oil, mixing thoroughly. Keep in the fridge where it will thicken further. Use flaxseed oil or cold-pressed sunflower seed oil if you are going to use all the dressing straight away as these are excellent oils for all the family.

# Salad Bowl

(V) [wf] [gf]

Little children will love to help you prepare this salad. I often find that most of the pepper has already been eaten before it goes in the salad bowl! Serve this with Salad Dressing page 156, and a baked potato. Use organic vegetables where possible.

  1 cos lettuce, shredded
  1 red pepper, deseeded and diced
  ½ cucumber, diced
  1 × 200 g (7 oz) tin of sweetcorn (no sugar, no salt) (optional)
  2 sticks celery, chopped
  2 tablespoons grated cheese
  a handful of raisins
  a handful of sprouted beans and seeds (pages 38–40)
  a handful of pumpkin and sunflower seeds

Throw all the ingredients together into a bowl and serve.

---

### Suggestions
You could also add diced chicken, flaked tuna or hard-boiled eggs to ring the changes and provide a salad main dish.

## Salad platters

It's good to get into the habit of producing platters of food for your children at an early age. Even if they start off not liking salad it allows them to make choices for themselves which they will enjoy. Experiment with a wide choice of colours and textures. Here are a few ideas:

- celery and/or carrot sticks
- cherry tomatoes
- red and/or yellow pepper slices
- mange tout
- radishes
- cucumber slices
- sprouted beans and seeds (pages 38–40)
- a small pile of raisins in the middle

# Beetroot and Carrot Salad

Ⓥ Ⓥ wf df gf

Serve this as an accompaniment to baked potatoes and Hummus (page 178). It is a lovely combination, and so colourful.

1 large raw beetroot
1 large carrot
a handful of raisins
25 g (1 oz) chopped walnuts (optional)
1 tablespoon Salad Dressing
1 tablespoon sesame seeds

Peel the raw beetroot and grate finely. Peel and grate the carrot and mix the two together. Add the raisins, walnuts if using, and dressing and sprinkle with the sesame seeds.

# Meat Dishes

## Chicken Parcels

wf df gf

My sister often used to cook me this when I went round to her house for a quick supper. I loved it then and my children love it now. The name 'chicken parcels' comes from the days when we cooked it wrapped in aluminium foil. However, aluminium is a heavy metal which does carry health risks and so it is no longer advisable to cook food directly on foil.

3 chicken quarters (or chicken thighs if you are only cooking for
   children)
For each chicken piece:
a few slices of onion
1/4 green pepper, thinly sliced
1 button mushroom, thinly sliced
1 clove garlic, peeled and crushed (optional)
some grated ginger
1 tablespoon tamari soy sauce (wheat-free)
1 tablespoon filtered water

Preheat the oven to 190°C/375°F/Gas Mark 5.

Place each chicken quarter (or thigh) in an ovenproof dish. Place the onion on top of the chicken. Then add the rest of the ingredients, piling them up on top. Grate over a little fresh ginger and pour over the soy sauce and the water.

Cover the chicken and place in the oven for 45 minutes (longer if you are doing lots) until cooked through. Take the chicken off the bone before serving.

# Chicken Fingers

df

These are so easy to prepare and free from any artificial flavours, colours or preservatives.

2 small boneless chicken breasts
4 tablespoons plain flour
2 organic eggs, beaten
2 slices wholemeal bread, made into breadcrumbs
extra-virgin olive oil or butter (for frying)

Slice the chicken breast into strips. Then prepare three shallow dishes: one with flour, one with beaten egg, and one with breadcrumbs. Roll the chicken strips in the flour first, then the egg and finally in the breadcrumbs until well coated.

Fry gently in a little olive oil or butter, turning occasionally, for 15 minutes or until cooked through.

# Steamed Roast Chicken

wf df gf

This is a much healthier way of roasting a chicken for all the family than covering the bird in flour, salt, oil or lard. The stock effectively steams the flesh which makes the meat more tender and gives it a better flavour.

1 organic chicken
1 onion
150 ml (5 fl oz) low-salt Marigold Swiss vegetable bouillon

Preheat the oven to 190°C/375°F/Gas Mark 5.

Place the chicken in a roasting dish, stuff with a peeled whole onion and pour the stock over the top. Roast for 1 hour, depending on weight, removing the lid after 35 minutes to brown the top. Baste the chicken with the stock when you remove the lid.

# Chicken Stew*

wf df gf

This is a great recipe for using up leftovers. Serve it with brown rice.

    2 tablespoons extra-virgin olive oil
    1 onion, peeled and chopped
    1 carrot, peeled and diced
    1 courgette, diced
    4–6 mushrooms, wiped and chopped
    1 × 400 g (14 oz) tin chopped tomatoes (no sugar, no salt)
    chicken leftovers, de-skinned and de-boned, chopped into small
        pieces (or 2 skinless, boneless chicken breasts)
    1 tablespoon chopped parsley

Heat the oil in a large pan and sauté the onion until transparent. Add the vegetables, tomatoes and chicken and simmer until the vegetables are cooked. Add the parsley and serve.

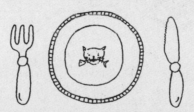

# Sticky Chicken

wf df gf

This is a rather sinful, and extremely messy way of eating chicken. It will suit children over the ages of three or four, once you are happy for them to chew off a bone! For younger children, you can take the chicken off the bone before serving. It's good with brown rice and stir-fried vegetables (see Chinese Stir-Fry, page 150).

> 10 organic chicken wings (or thighs)
> 2 cloves garlic, peeled and crushed
> 2.5 cm (1 in) piece of root ginger, finely chopped
> juice of 1 lemon
> 30 ml (1 fl oz) tamari soy sauce (wheat-free)
> 30 ml (1 fl oz) cold-pressed runny honey

Put the chicken wings or thighs into a shallow ovenproof dish and cover with the rest of the ingredients. Leave to marinate for 30 minutes, turning occasionally.

Bake in the oven, at 190°C/375°F/Gas Mark 5, for 30 minutes, turning and basting halfway through. The chicken will be cooked through and glazed with a delicious sticky sauce.

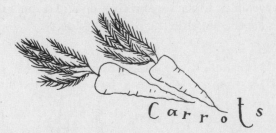

Carrots

# Classic Lamb Stew*

wf df gf

I love dishes that are quick to prepare and then involve a long, slow cooking time. You can get so much done in the meantime, without that last-minute panic when the children get back from school ravenously hungry. Remember, however, that red meat (beef, lamb, pork) should only be given to children once a week, as it is very high in saturated fat.

900 g (2 lb) stewing lamb (e.g. neck fillet)
3 cloves garlic, peeled and chopped
1 large onion, peeled and chopped
1 tablespoon extra-virgin olive oil
a large splash of red wine (optional)
850 ml (1½ pints) low-salt Marigold Swiss vegetable bouillon
2 large carrots, peeled and chopped
1 large parsnip, peeled and chopped
2 tablespoons potato flour or rice flour

Preheat the oven to 190°C/375°F/Gas Mark 5.

Cut the lamb into bite-size chunks, cutting off any excess fat. Using a large, heavy casserole dish, sauté the garlic and onion in the olive oil. Add the meat and brown it. Splash in the red wine if using, and cook for 2–3 minutes. Add the stock and vegetables. Mix the flour with a little cold water to prevent lumps and pour in, stirring well.

Cover the casserole and place in the oven. Turn the oven down to 150°C/300°F/Gas Mark 2 and cook for 2–3 hours. Keep checking that there is sufficient fluid and add a little more stock if necessary.

# Liver Casserole*

wf df gf

I know many parents do not like preparing liver, but it is the richest source of iron you can give your children. Only ever use organic liver as non-organic lamb's liver carries residues from any drugs and chemicals that the animal has been exposed to. As liver is a red meat, and high in vitamin A, limit it to once every other week. If you are not avoiding wheat, this recipe is delicious served on a bed of frilly pasta (like fiorelli) and sprinkled with chopped parsley.

Serve this casserole with mashed potato and a green vegetable.

1 large onion, peeled and chopped
2 tablespoons extra-virgin olive oil
4 slices organic lamb's liver
1 carrot, peeled and grated
1 red pepper, deseeded and chopped
1 green pepper, deseeded and chopped
1 dessertspoon potato flour mixed with a little cold water to prevent any lumps
200 ml (7 fl oz) low-salt Marigold Swiss vegetable bouillon
a generous splash of red wine (optional)

Sauté the onion in the oil in a frying pan until transparent. Add the liver and continue cooking for 5–10 minutes until the liver is cooked through and the juices run clear (if you pierce the chunks with a knife). Add the grated carrot and chopped peppers and sauté for 2–3 minutes. Add the potato flour and the stock, and the red wine if using and continue simmering for 10 minutes and serve.

# Healthy Lamb Burgers

df

These healthy lamb burgers make excellent substitutes for the heavily fat-laden hamburgers and beefburgers sold in supermarkets. They are extremely quick to make and an excellent recipe for a summer's Sunday lunch in the garden. Serve them on open wholemeal baps or in mini pitta breads with salad and sugar-free tomato ketchup.

1 medium courgette
1 small carrot, peeled
1 small onion, peeled
½ red pepper, deseeded
1 small ripe tomato
225 g (8 oz) organic lean minced lamb
1 organic egg, beaten
a handful of chopped parsley or mint
½ cup of wholemeal breadcrumbs
1 tablespoon extra-virgin olive oil

Roughly chop all the vegetables and tomato in a food processor and add them to the meat. Using your hands, mix in the beaten egg, parsley and breadcrumbs. Form into small burgers and fry in olive oil for 5–6 minutes on both sides.

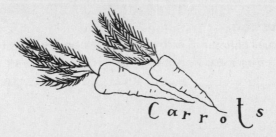

Carrots

# Vegetable Rich Mince*

wf  df  gf

Lamb is a much leaner meat to use than beef. Remember, however, that red meat (beef, lamb, pork) should only be given to children once a week, as it is very high in saturated fat.

You could also be adventurous and try some game mince like venison. Venison is rich in iron and low in saturated fat. You can now buy venison in supermarkets, but it is quite expensive.

1 large or 2 small onions, peeled and chopped
1 clove garlic, peeled and crushed
1 tablespoon olive oil
450 g (1 lb) lean lamb mince or venison mince
½ green pepper, deseeded and chopped
1 courgette, diced
a handful of mushrooms, finely chopped
1 carrot, peeled and diced
1 × 400 g (14 oz) can tomatoes (no sugar, no salt)
1 tablespoon tomato purée

Gently sauté the onion and garlic in the olive oil until translucent. Add the mince and brown well. Pour off any excess fat. Now add the rest of the ingredients and simmer for 1 hour, stirring occasionally. Ladle out any excess fat still remaining.

> **Suggestion**
> Add a cube of frozen spinach purée (if you have any in the freezer) to boost the mineral content even further.

# Gem Squash Surprise

wf df gf

This is a fun dish and incredibly easy to prepare. Remember, however, that red meat (beef, lamb, pork) should only be given to children once a week, as it is very high in saturated fat.

4 gem squash
8 tablespoons Vegetable Rich Mince (see opposite)

Preheat the oven to 190°C/375°F/Gas Mark 5.

Cut the top off each gem squash and scoop out the seeds. Fill each cavity with mince and pop the lids back on. Place the squashes in a deep oiled baking tray and cover with foil. If you are cooking two squashes, try placing them in a loaf tin – to stop them falling over.

Bake for 30 minutes until the flesh is soft. Allow to cool, and serve. Older children can eat them like boiled eggs. Scoop out the flesh for little ones.

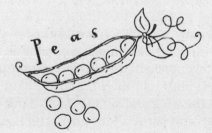

# Hearty Winter Stew*

$\boxed{\text{wf}}$ $\boxed{\text{df}}$ $\boxed{\text{gf}}$

I am very much in favour of supporting organic farms and I have therefore included this beef recipe. There has never been a case of BSE on an organic farm, where the cows have been born and raised on the farm itself. Remember, however, that red meat (beef, lamb, pork) should only be given to children once a week, as it is very high in saturated fat.

Serve this casserole with mashed potato or a baked potato and a green vegetable.

450 g (1 lb) organic beef casserole steak
1 large or 2 small onions
1 tablespoon extra-virgin olive oil
a generous splash of red wine (optional)
850 ml (1½ pints) low-salt Marigold Swiss vegetable bouillon
2 large carrots, peeled and chopped
1 parsnip, peeled and chopped
a handful of chopped parsley
2 heaped teaspoons potato flour

Preheat the oven to 190°C/375°F/Gas Mark 5.

Cut the beef into bite-size chunks, trimming off any excess fat (or ask your butcher to do it). In a heavy casserole dish, sauté the onions in the oil until translucent. Add the meat and brown it well. Throw in the wine and simmer for 2–3 minutes. Add the stock, vegetables and parsley. Mix the potato flour with a little cold water and stir in well.

Turn the oven down to 170°C/325°F/Gas Mark 3 and put the casserole in the oven for 2–3 hours until the meat is really tender. Keep checking that there is sufficient fluid.

# Fish Dishes

## Tuna Pasta Bake

wf df gf

1 clove garlic, peeled and chopped
1 large onion, peeled and chopped
1 tablespoon extra-virgin olive oil
½ red pepper, deseeded and chopped
½ yellow pepper, deseeded and chopped
1 courgette, diced
1 × 400 g (14 oz) tin chopped tomatoes (no sugar, no salt)
100 g (4 oz) dried rice pasta shapes or alternative wheat-free pasta
1 × 200 g (7 oz) tin of tuna (canned in water or oil, not brine)
grated Cheddar cheese

Sauté the garlic and onion in the oil for 5 minutes until transparent. Add the rest of the vegetables and tomatoes and simmer for approx. 15 minutes until cooked.

Cook the pasta separately. Drain the pasta and mix in the tuna and vegetable mixture. Pour into an ovenproof dish and sprinkle some grated cheese on top. Bake in the oven for 15–30 minutes before serving.

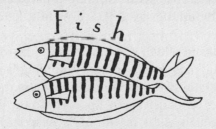

# Fish Pie*

By adding some oily fish like mackerel, herring or even salmon, you are including a rich source of the omega 3 essential fatty acids which are so important for growing children. Combined with the white fish, they won't even notice the difference. Once the children are over two years old, you can add some shellfish like shrimp and scallops. For those on wheat- and dairy-free diets, use the substitutes suggested. Serve with steamed broccoli and carrots.

1 large fillet of cod, haddock or coley
300 ml (10 fl oz) whole milk or unsweetened soya milk
1 fresh mackerel (without its head or tail) or 1 tin mackerel
    fillets in oil
some fresh herbs (e.g. parsley, tarragon, dill or chervil)
2 organic eggs
450 g (1 lb) potatoes, boiled and mashed

*White sauce*
1 tablespoon butter or unhydrogenated cooking margarine
2 tablespoons plain flour or 'All Purpose' flour
the milk in which the white fish was cooked
1 tablespoon chopped parsley

Preheat the oven to 190°C/375°F/Gas Mark 5.

Poach the fillet of fish in the milk for 20–30 minutes. If using fresh mackerel, stuff it with some fresh herbs and bake in the oven for 20–30 minutes as well. Meanwhile, hard-boil the two eggs.

Keep the milk in which you have cooked the white fish. Flake the fish carefully and put it in an ovenproof dish, making sure you remove all the skin and bones. Now make the white sauce. Heat the butter or margarine in a pan, stir in the flour to make a roux, and gradually beat in the milk. Keep stirring until you have a smooth sauce and then add the parsley. Chop up the eggs and add to the fish.

Make the sauce and pour over the fish and cover with the mashed potato. Bake in the oven for 30 minutes.

# Fish Fingers

[df]

These take very little time to prepare and are free from artificial colours, flavours or preservatives.

2 × 100 g (4 oz) portions of frozen coley, cod or haddock
4 tablespoons plain flour
2 organic eggs, beaten
2 slices wholemeal bread, made into breadcrumbs
extra-virgin olive oil or butter (for frying)

Defrost the fish and carefully cut each portion into five strips (ten in total). Prepare three shallow dishes: one with flour, one with the beaten egg, and one with the breadcrumbs. Roll the fish strips in the flour first, then the egg and finally in the bread-crumbs until well coated.

Fry in a little olive oil or butter, turning occasionally, for 15 minutes or until cooked through.

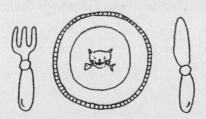

# Fishy Rice

wf | df | gf

This is an excellent storecupboard recipe when the fridge is empty! You could equally well use a fresh salmon fillet but you would need to bake it and check for bones first before adding it to the recipe. Purée for babies.

1 cup of brown rice
1 large onion, peeled and chopped
1 tablespoon extra-virgin olive oil
1 × 200 g (7 oz) tin wild red salmon or tuna (in water or oil, not brine)
1 × 200 g (7 oz) tin sweetcorn (no sugar, no salt)
a handful of chopped parsley
a little butter or unhydrogenated margarine

Wash the rice thoroughly and cook in a pan of boiling water for 25–30 minutes until cooked.

Meanwhile, sauté the onion in the oil until transparent. Put the onion in an ovenproof dish. Add the cooked rice, salmon or tuna, sweetcorn and parsley. Dot with butter or unhydrogenated margarine and heat in the oven for 20 minutes, at 160°C/325°F/ Gas Mark 3, before serving.

## Suggestion
If your child does not like sweetcorn then substitute a few frozen peas.

# Salmon Fishcakes

wf df gf

These are a family favourite and so easy to make.

200 g (7 oz) salmon fillet or 1 × 200 g (7 oz) tin wild red salmon
4 medium potatoes
1 medium onion, peeled and finely chopped
a little extra-virgin olive oil
1 organic egg, beaten
2 tablespoons chopped parsley
extra-virgin olive oil or butter (for frying)

If using fresh salmon, bake or steam it for 20 minutes until cooked. Peel and chop the potatoes, boil for 20 minutes (or until soft), and mash. Sauté the onion in a little olive oil for a few minutes until transparent.

In a large bowl, mix all the ingredients together and form eight small or four large fishcakes. Place in the fridge for 1 hour before cooking to firm them up. Gently fry in extra-virgin olive oil or butter until crisp on both sides.

> **Suggestion**
> You could replace the salmon with other fish like cod, tuna, haddock or coley.

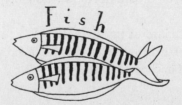

# Salmon Pesto Spaghetti

df

This strange combination works really well. The red pesto has a delicious flavour and its addition will encourage even an ardent fish-hater to try this dish! Serve it with a salad or steamed broccoli florets.

> 2 × 250 g (9 oz) skinless and boneless salmon fillets
> ½ packet wholemeal spaghetti
> a splash of extra-virgin olive oil
> 1 tablespoon good-quality red pesto

Preheat the oven to 190°C/375°F/Gas Mark 5, and bake the salmon for 20 minutes until cooked. Flake and remove any bones. Cook the pasta, drain and drizzle with olive oil. Add the flaked salmon and red pesto, mix well and serve.

# Instant Fishy Pasta Sauce

df

This is a really quick storecupboard dish, rich in essential fatty acids. By adding sweetcorn and tomato ketchup, you can subdue the strong taste of the fish. Serve with pasta shapes.

> 1 × 125 g (5 oz) tin of sardines in tomato sauce or pilchards in tomato sauce
> 2 tablespoons sugar-free tomato ketchup
> 1 × 200 g (7 oz) tin of sweetcorn (no sugar, no salt)
> a small handful of chopped flatleaf parsley

Mash the sardines or pilchards with the tomato ketchup. Add the sweetcorn and flatleaf parsley. Mix up well with the pasta and serve.

# Fish Stew

wf df gf

This recipe is packed with trace elements, especially iron and zinc. Serve it with green beans or broccoli and hot soda bread or mashed potato. For children over two and adults, you can add shellfish (which is an excellent source of zinc and calcium). Prawns, scallops and clams go really well in this dish.

1 medium onion, peeled and chopped
1 garlic clove, peeled and finely chopped
1 tablespoon extra-virgin olive oil
1 × 450 g (1 lb) mixed seafood (cod fillet, salmon fillet, prawns, scallops, clams, mussels, etc)
1 tablespoon chopped flatleaf parsley
1 carrot, sliced
250 ml (9 fl oz) low-salt Marigold Swiss vegetable bouillon
2 tablespoons white wine
2 ripe tomatoes
1 tablespoon tomato purée
a bay leaf
a handful of chopped parsley

In a large pot, sauté the onion and garlic in the olive oil until the onion is transparent. Add the mixed seafood and the flatleaf parsley and sauté for another 5 minutes. Add the carrot, stock, wine, tomatoes, tomato purée and then the bay leaf. Bring to the boil and then simmer gently for 25–30 minutes. Sprinkle with parsley and serve.

# Grilled Sardine and Cheese Toasties

This is a variation on the previous recipe.

1 quantity Instant Fishy Pasta Sauce (see page 174)
4 pieces wholemeal or rye bread
grated organic Cheddar cheese or soya cheese

Make the Instant Fishy Pasta Sauce. Toast the bread lightly, pile the sardine mixture on the toast, sprinkle lightly with cheese and pop under the grill for a couple of minutes.

# Salmon Parcels

df

This is a variation on the previous recipe. If your child is avoiding wheat, you can buy rice sheets at Thai supermarkets. Again, you could use any fish. Serve with a selection of green vegetables.

2 sheets of filo pastry or rice paper per fillet
a little olive oil (for brushing)
a little chopped spring onion
a little chopped coriander
3 skinless and boneless salmon fillets
poppy seeds (for decoration)

Preheat the oven to 190°C/375°F/Gas Mark 5.
Carefully brush the sheets of filo pastry or rice paper with olive oil and place carefully one on top of the other. Place the spring onion and coriander on top of the fillets. Then put the fillet at one end of the filo pastry. Fold the end over the fillet, then

tuck the sides in, and roll the fillet along the length of the phyllo pastry.

Bake on a baking tray for 20–25 minutes until cooked. Allow to cool a little before serving and sprinkle with poppy seeds for decoration if you wish.

# Baked Sea Bass

wf df gf

This sounds like a terribly adult recipe but it was a hit in our household. I introduced my boys to coriander very early on, as I love it. I recommend that you scrape off all the herbs the first time you serve it, as the flavours can be a bit strong in isolation. You can use this combination to brighten up even the most boring of white fish.

Serve with mashed potato and green vegetables. It is also particularly good on a bed of pak choi and brown rice, and it can be puréed for babies.

    4 skinless and boneless fillets of sea bass
    2 garlic cloves, peeled and crushed
    a little chopped coriander
    a little grated ginger
    1 small spring onion, finely chopped
    a small knob of butter or unhydrogenated margarine

Preheat the oven to 190°C/375°F/Gas Mark 5.

Place the fillets of sea bass in a glass ovenproof container and pop all the other ingredients on top. Cover and cook for 20–30 minutes, depending on how many fillets you are cooking.

# Dips and Spreads

## Hummus

(V) wf df gf

Hummus is such a versatile food. You can use it as a dip or a quick snack on a cracker or piece of toast. Or, for a baby over nine months, you can mash it up in a baked potato or add it to vegetable purées. It keeps well in the fridge for three to five days.

**MAKES ABOUT 450 G (1 LB)**

1 × 400 g (14 oz) can chickpeas (no sugar, no salt)
2 tablespoons tahini
2 tablespoons fresh lemon juice
1 tablespoon olive oil
1 garlic clove, peeled

Put all the ingredients into a food processor and blend until smooth and creamy.

## Peanut Butter Dip

(V) wf gf

If your children like peanut butter, they will love this dip. It's best eaten the same day.

**MAKES ABOUT 3 TABLESPOONS**

2 tablespoons smooth peanut butter
1 tablespoon creamy live yogurt
a pinch of cumin
a squeeze of lemon juice

Stir all the ingredients together in a bowl.

# Avocado Dip

Ⓥ

This makes a lovely creamy dip. Adding a few drops of hot tabasco makes it more interesting as an adult dip.

### MAKES ABOUT 8 TABLESPOONS

1 small ripe avocado
a squeeze of fresh lemon juice (to prevent browning)
1 garlic clove, peeled
2 tablespoons live yogurt or cream cheese
1 tablespoon organic sugar-free tomato ketchup

Blend all the ingredients in a food processor until smooth. This dip does not keep longer than a day in the fridge.

# Guacamole

Ⓥ ● wf df gf

This rustic dip will appeal to the more adventurous toddler appetite. It's best eaten straight away, as it goes brown if left in the fridge.

### MAKES ABOUT 8 TABLESPOONS

1 ripe avocado
1 tablespoon fresh lemon juice
1 spring onion
1 garlic clove, peeled
2 very ripe tomatoes

Roughly chop all the ingredients together in a food processor and serve immediately.

# Veg and Nut Pâté

(V) (V) [wf] [df] [gf]

This is another really versatile dish – it keeps for about five days in the fridge. You could serve it as a spread on oatcakes, rice cakes, rye crackers or toast, or use it as a dip with fresh vegetables and salt-free corn chips. For a younger baby, you could serve it mixed with rice, millet or mashed into a baked potato or sweet potato (from nine months). Any variety of vegetables and nuts works well.

    50 g (2 oz) celery
    75 g (3 oz) carrots
    50 g (2 oz) leeks
    50 g (2 oz) onions
    a handful of chopped coriander
    a few mushrooms
    1 garlic clove, peeled
    50 g (2 oz) sunflower seeds, ground
    50 g (2 oz) hazelnuts, ground
    a little black pepper
    a little Marigold Swiss low-salt vegetable bouillon (optional)

Peel, wash and chop the vegetables. Then steam them until soft. Add the garlic, and purée in a food processor and mix with the ground seeds and nuts. Season with pepper and bouillon powder (if necessary) and chill before serving.

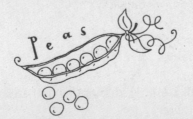

# Home-made Smooth Nut Butters

(V) (V) [wf] [df] [gf]

These are very easy to make and free from sugar, salt and palm oil. You can use a combination of different nuts or just one type at a time. Keep nut butters in the fridge for two to three weeks.

> 250 g (9 oz) nuts (e.g. almonds, walnuts, cashews, peanuts, hazelnuts)
> 2 heaped tablespoons sun-dried raisins
> a little olive oil or walnut oil

Lightly roast the nuts in the oven. (Don't forget them – as I have, so many times!)

Place the nuts and raisins in a food processor and mix to a smooth paste. This will take some time. Add some oil, a little at a time, if needed to get the right consistency. It will depend on the type of nuts.

---

### Suggestion

You can also make seed butters using the same method. Use sunflower or pumpkin for best results. However, it is much easier to buy tahini (pulped sesame seeds), as they are so small to grind.

---

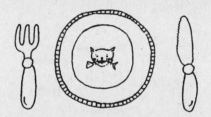

# Baking

## Soda Bread

Ⓥ

There is nothing quite like a hunk of warm soda bread thickly spread with hummus or nut butter. Soda bread is nicest eaten the day it's made, but it can be toasted the following day to revive it!

### MAKES 1 LOAF

450 g (1 lb) plain wholemeal and unbleached white flour, mixed
2 teaspoons bicarbonate of soda
25 g (1 oz) butter or unhydrogenated vegetable margarine
300 ml (10 fl oz) buttermilk or natural yogurt

Preheat the oven to 190°C/375°F/Gas Mark 5.

Sift the flour and bicarbonate of soda into a mixing bowl. Add the butter or margarine and rub in until it resembles fine bread-crumbs. Make a well in the centre and add the buttermilk or yogurt. Mix together into a dough. Turn the dough out onto a floured board and knead it into a round loaf.

Put onto a non-stick baking tray and cut a criss-cross in the top. Bake for 30 minutes until it has risen and is golden-brown and crusty. Cool on a wire rack and preferably eat the same day or as toast the following day.

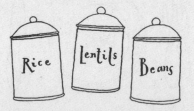

# Oatcake Animals or Fingers

(V) (V) wf df gf

These are a great accompaniment to soups or dips, or they make a convenient snack accompanied by some fruit or a slice of organic Cheddar or soya cheese.

**MAKES ABOUT 15 ANIMALS**

225 g (8 oz) fine oatmeal
a pinch of bicarbonate of soda
1 tablespoon sunflower oil
6 tablespoons boiling filtered water

Put the oatmeal in a bowl and add the bicarbonate of soda through a sieve to guarantee even distribution. Mix the oil and water together and add slowly to make a stiff dough. Leave for a few minutes to allow to swell.

Roll out thinly, on a surface dusted with oatmeal, and cut into animal shapes. We use the play dough cutters! Alternatively, you can just cut it into fingers. Place on a baking tray and bake at 180°C/350°F/Gas Mark 4 for 25 minutes. Do not allow to brown.

Store in an airtight container. They should keep for about a week.

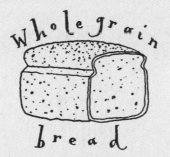

# Almond Biscuits

(V) [df]

This is a perfect recipe for your family to make with you. All children love cooking and being creative. We usually make these around Christmas time, using star and Christmas tree cutters.

**MAKES ABOUT 20 BISCUITS**

100 g (4 oz) ground almonds
225 g (8 oz) wholewheat flour
2 tablespoons fructose (fruit sugar) or maple syrup
a pinch of salt
175 g (6 oz) unhydrogenated margarine or butter
2 egg yolks

Preheat the oven to 190°C/375°F/Gas Mark 5.

In a bowl, mix the almonds, flour, fructose or maple syrup and salt. Melt the margarine or butter in a pan over a low heat, let it cool a little, then beat in the egg yolks. Mix the wet and dry ingredients together to form a stiff dough. You may find it a bit crumbly, so use your hands.

Roll out carefully on a floured surface and use cutters to form shapes. Place on a well-greased baking tray and bake in the oven for 10–15 minutes.

# Puddings

I'm not a huge fan of puddings because they tend to increase a child's daily sugar consumption dramatically and can encourage fussy eating. Fruit is naturally sweet – a perfect pudding. By avoiding sweet puddings, you will help your child maintain his energy levels and avoid the tiredness, irritability, mood swings and hyperactive behaviour commonly associated with high sugar intake. However, even I have to admit that there is nothing more delicious than a bowl of apple crumble and custard on a cold winter's day! Here's a mixture of mainly sugar-free recipes for those who love their puddings!

## Fruit Smoothie

(V) (V) [wf] [df] [gf]

These are a delicious alternative pudding to yogurt and they ensure an excellent vitamin intake. Suitable for all age groups.

**SERVES 1 CHILD**

1 banana
½ mango

Peel and roughly chop the fruit. Then whizz in a food processor until smooth and serve.

> **Suggestions**
> Try other combinations of fruit like peaches, strawberries, pawpaw, or kiwi. If you want a creamy consistency, using banana as a base is a good idea. Add some natural yogurt and some milk and you have a delicious fruity milkshake.

# Tropical Fruit Salad

Ⓥ Ⓥ wf gf

When I introduced this fruit salad to my children, we used to play guessing games to see if we could guess what fruit the boys had in their mouths. They then had to tell us what it really was and we inevitably ended up with uncontrollable giggles! Include the orange juice for children of a year and over. Serve with creamy natural yogurt.

**SERVES 2 ADULTS AND 2 CHILDREN**

1 banana
½ mango
½ cantaloupe melon
1 kiwi fruit
1 apple
1 slice of pineapple
juice of 1–2 oranges (optional)

Make sure all the fruit is really ripe and therefore lovely and sweet rather than sour! Peel and chop the fruit into bite-size pieces, mix together in a bowl and serve.

## Fresh fruit platters

A platter of fresh fruit makes a wonderfully refreshing pudding. Like a Salad Platter (page 158), it encourages your children to be adventurous and make choices for themselves. They can enjoy this at any age.

- apple slices
- pear slices
- pineapple slices, cut into quarters
- grapes, whole or halved
- strawberries, whole or quartered
- banana chunks
- melon balls
- satsuma segments

# Mango Hedgehog

(V) (V) [wf] [df] [gf]

Children can enjoy these at any age.

**1 MANGO MAKES 2 HEDGEHOGS**

1 mango

Slice the mango in half down one side of its stone. Lay one half on its back on a chopping board. Cut the flesh into a 'noughts and crosses' shape, leaving the skin intact. Fold inside out and it looks like a hedgehog. Children can then eat it with their fingers.

# Fruit Bugs

(V) (V) [wf] [df] [gf]

This inspired idea was given to me by a New Zealand nanny called Fiona. She called them 'Doodlebugs'. Even children who are not that keen on fruit will enjoy making these.

**SERVES 1 CHILD**

½ orange (per bug)
assortment of cubed fruit (e.g. apple, pear, kiwi, berries,
    grapes, etc)
cocktail sticks
a few raisins (optional)

Cut the orange in half and lay it down on its flat side. Stick the cubed fruit onto the cocktail sticks and push into the orange. We often use a couple of raisins for the eyes.

# Baked Apple with Molasses

Ⓥ Ⓥ wf df gf

The addition of molasses makes this age-old dessert rich in trace elements and wonderfully gooey. This recipe is also suitable from six months onwards. For a baby, you will need to scoop the cooked apple out of the skin. Serve with unsweetened or baked custard, natural live yogurt or a little appropriate milk.

### SERVES 1 CHILD

1 eating apple
a few sultanas (unglazed variety)
1 teaspoon crude blackstrap molasses (unsulphured)
apple juice or water (enough to cover the bottom of the ovenproof container)

Preheat the oven to 190°C/375°F/Gas Mark 5.

Core the apple and put it in a small ovenproof container. Fill the hole in the middle of the apple with sultanas and pour the molasses on top. Surround the apple with apple juice or water, cover and bake in the oven for 40 minutes or until soft.

# Fresh Custard

Ⓥ wf gf

Once you have made fresh custard, you will never go back to the packet version. Real custard is a creamy colour and free from all colours, flavours and preservatives. Serve it with fresh fruit salad, stewed apple or crumble. Cold custard is equally delicious but there is scarcely ever any left in our house!

This recipe works just as well with fortified soya milk as it does with whole milk. If you use soya milk that is slightly sweetened with apple juice concentrate, omit the maple syrup.

**MAKES 300 ML (10 FL OZ)**

2 large egg yolks
1 tablespoon maple syrup
1 heaped teaspoon cornflour or arrowroot
1 teaspoon vanilla extract
300 ml (10 fl oz) whole milk or enriched soya milk

In a heatproof bowl, beat the egg yolks, maple syrup, cornflour or arrowroot and vanilla extract together. Warm the milk and pour into the egg mixture. Mix together and return to the pan and stir over a low heat until the mixture coats the back of the spoon or reaches your desired consistency.

# Banana Custard

(V) [wf] [gf]

A perennial favourite. Again, you can make a dairy-free version if you use soya milk for the custard. You can make the custard in advance for this recipe but do not cut the banana up until just before serving or it will go brown.

**SERVES 2 ADULTS AND 2 CHILDREN**

4 bananas
600 ml (1 pint) Fresh Custard (see above)

Slice the bananas and put them in a bowl, pour over the custard and serve.

# Brown Rice Pudding

(V) [wf] [gf]

You can make this for babies under a year old if you use formula or breast milk instead of the milks suggested. Use soya milk if you want to make a dairy-free version.

**SERVES 2 CHILDREN**

100 g (4 oz) easy-cook brown rice
a handful of sun-dried raisins
600 ml (1 pint) whole milk or enriched soya milk

Grease an ovenproof dish. Wash the rice and sprinkle it on the bottom of the dish. Add the raisins and milk and bake in the oven for 2 hours at 150°C/300°F/Gas Mark 2.

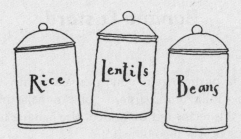

# Blueberry Semolina

Ⓥ

Semolina is made of soft wheat from which all the bran has been removed. It is therefore an excellent way to introduce wheat into a child's diet. Blueberries are naturally sweet, unlike some other berries, and so can be eaten raw. They are a good source of vitamin C and have anti-bacterial properties. They also contain anthocyanins (compounds which are particularly effective against some forms of E. coli bacteria, the main culprits in many tummy upsets).

Use soya milk for a dairy-free version.

**SERVES 1 CHILD**

150 ml (5 fl oz) whole milk or soya milk
2 heaped teaspoons semolina
a handful of blueberries, washed carefully and destalked

Put the milk into a saucepan and add the semolina. Heat gently, stirring all the time, for 5 minutes until the liquid thickens. Whizz up the blueberries in a food processor and pour into the semolina. An instant purple pudding!

## Suggestions

For older children, why not try adding a teaspoon of 100 per cent fruit jam (e.g. Meridian raspberry) to a serving of plain semolina – my boys love it. Alternatively, you can just add a couple of cubes of frozen fruit purée.

# Fresh Fruit Juice Jelly

(V) (V) wf df gf

Making your own jelly is as easy as making packet jelly. The benefits are that it is not full of sugar or artificial colours, as are most of the commercially produced jellies. You need to use some bright-coloured juices for the best effect (e.g. unsweetened pineapple juice or unsweetened orange juice if you are making the jelly for children of a year or over). Or you can use diluted juice concentrates like apple and blackcurrant (made only from juice, with no added sugar).

This recipe will make six small party jellies. If you use a 600 ml (1 pint) jelly mould, you could place fruit in the bottom (e.g. a selection of berries or some apple, banana and mandarin) and then pour the juice on top for a fresh fruit jelly.

**SERVES 6 CHILDREN**

600 ml (1 pint) fresh fruit juice or diluted juice concentrate
1 sachet vegegel or 1 teaspoon agar agar flakes

Heat 50 ml (2 fl oz) of the juice in a pan until nearly boiling, then sprinkle the gelatin equivalent over it. Stir until all the crystals have dissolved. Add this mixture to the rest of the juice, mixing thoroughly. Refrigerate until firm.

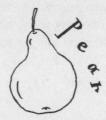

# Buckwheat Pancakes

Ⓥ

Buckwheat is a wonderfully versatile food. Traditionally, French crêpes were always made with buckwheat flour as it makes a lighter pancake. Buckwheat, despite its name, has nothing to do with wheat and is therefore a very good substitute for those on a wheat-free or gluten-free diet.

Use soya milk for a dairy-free version. And replace the whole-wheat flour with buckwheat flour for a wheat-free version.

Fill each pancake with fruit (e.g. mashed banana, apple purée, pear slices, mixed summer fruits, etc), top with natural live yogurt or fromage frais if desired, and sprinkle with chopped nuts and maple syrup for older children.

**SERVES 2 ADULTS AND 2 CHILDREN**

½ cup buckwheat flour and ½ cup wholewheat flour
2 organic eggs, beaten
1 cup whole milk or soya milk
a pinch of salt
a knob of butter or vegetarian margarine

In a bowl, mix the flour and eggs and slowly add the milk, stirring well to prevent lumps forming. (Mix the ingredients together in a food processor if you want.) Add a pinch of salt.

Heat a frying pan, add a knob of butter or margarine and put enough of the mixture in to coat the bottom of the pan. Cook both sides until dry. Stack the pancakes on top of each other.

# Apple Crumble*

(V) (V) [df]

This is my family's very favourite pudding in the world. I much prefer to stew the apple first; I think it gives the pudding a much nicer texture and you can get a really distinctive taste with the addition of the spices. If you use eating apples, you do not have to use any sweetener as they are naturally sweet.

When there was a baby in the house, I used to stew lots of apples all in one go to make apple purée and freeze them using the ice cube method (page 24). The ice cubes often ended up as my apple base for a crumble. A useful short cut!

**SERVES 2 ADULTS AND 2 CHILDREN**

a 1 kg (2 lb) bag of eating apples, peeled, cored and sliced
2 handfuls of sun-dried raisins or unsweetened sultanas
250 ml (9 fl oz) filtered water
4 cloves
a pinch of cinnamon

*Crumble*
100 g (4 oz) wholemeal flour
75 g (3 oz) butter or vegetarian margarine
40 g (1½ oz) light muscovado sugar
a handful of oats
2 tablespoons wheatgerm
2 tablespoons sesame seeds

Put the apples and raisins or sultanas in a pan and add the water, cloves and cinnamon. Cover and bring to the boil. Simmer for 20 minutes until soft and mushy. Remove the cloves once cooked. Transfer the apple mixture to an ovenproof dish!

To make the crumble, put the flour, butter or margarine, and sugar into a bowl. Rub together with your fingertips until the mixture resembles fine breadcrumbs and there are no lumps of butter left. Add the rest of the ingredients, mixing them in with your hands, and pour on top of your apple. Bake for 20–30 minutes, at 190°C/375°F/Gas Mark 5, until the crumble topping is crisp.

---

### Suggestions

You can substitute many other fruits for the apple. Plums, gooseberries, blackberry and apple, banana and mango (unusual and very delicious), rhubarb and pear all make excellent crumbles.

---

# Instant Chocolate Pudding

Ⓥ Ⓥ [wf] [df] [gf]

This is a dairy-free, high-protein pudding. I have no problem giving really good-quality chocolate to children once in a while. Never say never to a child – it is fatal!

**SERVES 1 CHILD**

1 ripe banana
½ × 225 g (8 oz) pack silken tofu
1 dessertspoon organic 70 per cent cocoa grated chocolate

Whizz all the ingredients up together in a food processor and serve with extra grated chocolate sprinkled on top.

# Yogurt Lollies

 (V) [wf] [gf]

**MAKES 4 YOGURT LOLLIES**

fruit juice concentrate
500 g (1lb 2 oz) creamy natural yogurt
lolly moulds

Pour enough fruit juice concentrate into a large pot of natural yogurt to get your desired colour and sweetness. Mix really well and pour into the lolly moulds. One large pot of yogurt will make four yogurt lollies. Freeze until set. To prevent pulling the sticks out without the lollies, run the moulds under hot water and leave for a few minutes before serving.

> ### Suggestion
> You can also use flavoured yogurts (e.g. Yeo Valley Organic Strawberry Yogurt) and then you do not have to use any natural sweeteners.

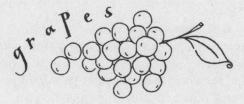

# Fruity Ice Lollies*

(V) (V) [wf] [df] [gf]

Perfect for a boiling hot summer day – ice lollies that are free of extra sugar and artificial colours and sweeteners. Every supermarket sells cheap lolly moulds during the summer months. You can either use fresh juice diluted half and half or use a diluted fruit juice concentrate.

apple and blackcurrant fruit juice concentrate
filtered water
lolly moulds

These fruit juice concentrates are very strong, so it is advisable to dilute them as recommended on the bottles. Freeze in the lolly moulds until set.

> ## Suggestion
> You can now buy fruit smoothies as drinks at some supermarkets and sandwich shops. These also make excellent ice lollies. But watch out for hidden sugar – make sure they're only made from fruit.

# Banana Ice Cream*

(V) [wf] [gf]

This only takes a couple of minutes to prepare and a couple of hours to freeze. Make sure you take it out of the freezer at the beginning of the meal to allow it to soften, as it tends to freeze rock solid!

If you are feeding lots of toddlers, it may be easier to freeze the ice cream using the ice cube method (page 24). Serve plain or with fresh banana, puréed raspberries or fruit compôte.

**MAKES ABOUT 600 ML (1 PINT)**

4 very ripe bananas
1 × 300 ml (10 fl oz) tub creamy natural yogurt (Yeo Valley is a good one)
juice of ½ lemon
1 teaspoon lecithin granules
1 tablespoon maple syrup
1 tablespoon tahini (ground sesame seeds)

Either mash up all the ingredients together or, alternatively, throw them all in a food processor and mix until smooth. Pour into a freezer container and freeze for a couple of hours or until firm.

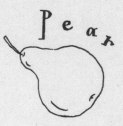

# Almond Fruit Tarts

(V) [df]

Here's another idea for dressing up fruit.

**MAKES 16–20 PASTRY CASES**

225 g (8 oz) wholemeal flour
100 g (4 oz) ground almonds
a pinch of salt
25 g (1 oz) muscovado sugar
175 g (6 oz) unhydrogenated margarine
1 organic egg, beaten
fresh fruit (e.g. strawberries, raspberries, or sliced apples or pears)
creamy natural yogurt
maple syrup

Preheat the oven to 190°C/375°F/Gas Mark 5.

Mix the flour, almonds, salt and sugar together in a bowl and rub in the margarine. Add the egg to form a soft dough. Roll out the pastry nice and thinly, cut into 16–20 circles, and put them into a well-greased tartlet tray. Bake for 15 minutes.

Allow to cool. Then fill each tart with fresh fruit, topped with creamy natural yogurt and a little drizzle of maple syrup.

---

**Suggestion**

For children's parties, you could fill these cases with 100 per cent fruit jam to make jam tarts.

---

# Sweet Treats and Party Food

## Banana Birthday Cake

Ⓥ

This was the first recipe that I ever put in one of my articles for *Natural Parent*. I have yet to find a parent or child who does not like this sugar-free cake. I often use it as a base for a birthday cake.

For a dairy-free version, use unhydrogenated margarine rather than butter.

**MAKES 8–10 GOOD SLICES**

100 g (4 oz) self-raising wholemeal flour (preferably organic)
½ teaspoon mixed spice
50 g (2 oz) butter or unhydrogenated margarine
75 g (3 oz) sun-dried raisins
225 g (8 oz) banana
1 organic egg, beaten

Preheat the oven to 180°C/350°F/Gas Mark 4.

Mix the flour and spice in a bowl. Rub in the butter or margarine and stir in the raisins. In a separate bowl, mash the banana and egg. Stir into the flour mixture and put into a well-greased rectangular loaf tin.

Turn the oven down to 160°C/325°F/Gas Mark 3 and cook on the middle shelf for 1 hour or until cooked.

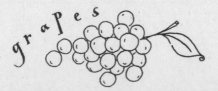

# Magical Muffins

(V) [df]

These sugar-free muffins are an excellent snack, pudding or even quick breakfast before school. They will keep well in a tin and are so popular that it is well worth making them in bulk. I often make them in double quantities.

**MAKES ABOUT 7 MUFFINS OR 15 IF USING FAIRY CAKE CASES**

225 g (8 oz) wholemeal self-raising flour
a pinch of ground cinnamon
a pinch of ground nutmeg
50 g (2 oz) chopped pecans
50 g (2 oz) desiccated coconut
175 g (6 oz) carrots, peeled and grated
175 g (6 oz) eating apples, peeled and grated
75 g (3 oz) chopped dates
2 small organic eggs, beaten
100 ml (4 fl oz) sunflower oil
1 teaspoon vanilla extract

Preheat the oven to 180°C/350°F/Gas Mark 4.

Mix all the dry ingredients together in one bowl and all the wet ingredients together in a separate bowl. Add the dry ingredients to the wet and mix thoroughly. Your children will love doing this with their hands – it is so sticky! Spoon into muffin cases and place on a baking tray. Bake for 18–20 minutes.

# Date Slices

Ⓥ Ⓥ

These wholesome biscuits are sugar-free and very easy to make. Use unhydrogenated margarine, rather than butter, for a dairy-free version.

**MAKES ABOUT 12 SLICES**

225 g (8 oz) pitted dates (not sugar-rolled)
50 ml (5 fl oz) filtered water
175 g (6 oz) spelt flour or plain wholemeal flour
175 g (6 oz) porridge oats
175 g (6 oz) butter or unhydrogenated margarine

Preheat the oven to 190°C/375°F/Gas Mark 5 and grease a small square baking tin.

Put the dates in a saucepan with 50 ml (5 fl oz) filtered water and simmer until the dates are soft and mushy. Whizz them in the blender until you get a smooth date purée. Put to one side to cool down.

Meanwhile, sift the flour into a bowl and add the oats and the butter or margarine. Rub the butter or margarine into the flour mixture and add 2–4 tablespoons filtered water to create a dough. Put half the dough into the greased tin and press it down flat. Place the date purée on top and smooth it out with a knife. Roll out the remaining dough and place on top, pressing down firmly.

Bake in the oven for half an hour. Leave to cool, then cut into small squares.

# Date and Nut Truffles

(V) (V) [wf] [df] [gf]

These will be adored by adults and children. Great as an occasional teatime treat or for a party.

**MAKES 12–15 TRUFFLES**

100 g (4 oz) unsalted cashews
4 tablespoons Date Purée (page 90)
desiccated coconut

Grind the cashews in a food processor or coffee grinder and put into a mixing bowl. Add 4 tablespoons Date Purée and mix thoroughly until smooth. Roll into little balls in your hand and cover in desiccated coconut. Put in the fridge for a couple of hours to set.

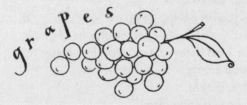

# Terri's Carrot Cake

(V)

This amazing recipe was given to me by a New Zealand nanny called Terri. She used to make this large version in my chicken roasting pan and it would all be gone within three days! However, you can just as easily make it as a sandwich cake, using two sponge cake tins and putting the icing in the middle. I have kept the measurements in cups in order to get it as close to her original as possible. It is very easy to get hold of measuring cups these days, as most supermarkets now sell them.

**MAKES 1 LARGE CAKE**

½ cup sunflower seeds
1 cup wholemeal flour
½ cup plain flour
1 cup rolled oats
2 teaspoons mixed spice
3 level teaspoons baking powder
100 g (4 oz) walnuts, chopped or blended lightly
500 g (1 lb 2 oz) dates soaked in boiling water to soften, drained and blended lightly
1 courgette, grated
2 carrots, peeled and grated
4 large organic eggs, beaten
2 cups sunflower oil
¼ cup maple syrup or dark muscavado sugar (optional)

*Icing*
400 g (14 oz) or 1½ cups cream cheese
icing sugar (as little as you can to make an icing)

Preheat the oven to 180°C/350°F/Gas Mark 4.
  Put all the cake ingredients into a bowl, except for the eggs,

the oil and the maple syrup. Using your hands, mix it all up together and then add the remaining ingredients. Children love helping with this bit, as it is so mucky!

Put the mixture in a large greased cake tin and bake for 1 hour. If still doughy after an hour, turn the oven off, cover with tin foil and leave the cake in the oven for another half an hour. The gooier the better!

# Popcorn

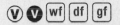

Most children love to hear popcorn being made, especially if they see the kernels first – it can be mummy's magic trick! We always have popcorn plain without salt or sugar and the children love it. Alternatively, you can drizzle a teaspoon of molasses over the top to increase the nutrient value.

**SERVES 2 ADULTS AND 2 CHILDREN**

2 tablespoons olive oil
4 tablespoons popcorn kernels

Heat the oil in a deep saucepan so that it goes runny and coats the bottom of the pan. Add the popcorn and put the lid on. After a few minutes the corn will start to pop.

When the popping slows down, it should be done.

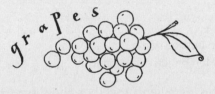

# Drinks

## Apple and Carrot Juice

(V) (V) [wf] [df] [gf]

This is a really good drink when there are coughs and colds in the house as the carrots are full of beta-carotene (the precursor to vitamin A) which helps strengthen the mucus membranes.

**SERVES 1 CHILD**

½ carrot, peeled
½ apple, peeled and cored
a little filtered water

Put the carrot and apple through a juicer and dilute with a little filtered water. Serve straight away.

## Banana Milk

(V) (V) [wf] [df] [gf]

My eldest loved this as he was getting used to a feeder cup. Using a little lemon juice will prevent the banana turning brown so quickly. Avoid using unripe bananas which are acid-forming and can cause constipation. When a banana ripens, the starches change into sugars and are more digestible.

**SERVES 1 CHILD**

1 ripe banana
1 cup filtered bottled water
a squeeze of lemon juice (optional)

Liquidise all the ingredients together and serve straight away.

# Tangerine and Banana Juice

(V) (V) [wf] [df] [gf]

This is so delicious. You will get the best results if you have a juicer (you can buy really cheap ones now at good department stores). Bananas don't really juice but the result is a creamy mixture that children love.

**SERVES 1 CHILD**

1 banana
1 tangerine

Peel the fruit, put through a juicer and serve straight away.

# Banana and Almond Shake Supreme

(V) (V) [wf] [df] [gf]

A milk-free milkshake!

**SERVES 2 CHILDREN**

1 cup of Almond Milk (see previous recipe)
2 frozen bananas, roughly chopped
a pinch of ground nutmeg or cinnamon

Put the Almond Milk into a food processor or liquidiser and slowly add the bananas in order to reach the desired thickness and avoid lumps being left unblended.

Add the nutmeg or cinnamon and serve.

# Almond Milk

Ⓥ Ⓥ ⌊wf⌋ ⌊df⌋ ⌊gf⌋

Almond milk is more of an acquired taste, I find. Some children love it, some don't. But it is so full of goodness that it's worth trying it out on the family two or three times to get them hooked. It is an excellent source of protein, calcium and magnesium (all needed by growing children). You can adjust the quantity of nuts, depending on your desired thickness, but the general rule for nut and seed milks is to use 1 part nut or seed to 3 parts water. Almond milk will keep in the fridge for a couple of days. If you want to blanch your own almonds, put them in a sieve and dip them in a pan of boiling water for 30 seconds – the skins will then pop off very easily.

**MAKES ABOUT 600 ML (1 PINT)**

¼ cup blanched almonds
1 cup filtered water
a pinch of ground cinnamon or nutmeg
a little cold-pressed honey (optional)

Place the blanched almonds and the water in a food processor and blend until the mixture becomes thick and smooth (a couple of minutes). Strain the liquid through a fine sieve or piece of cheesecloth to remove the pulp. If there is a great deal of pulp you can repeat the process. Add the cinnamon or nutmeg and sweeten to taste with a little honey if necessary. This milk does tend to separate, so you will need to stir it before serving.

# Energy Shake

(V) (V) [wf] [df] [gf]

I love this for my breakfast. It is a meal in itself – full of protein, vitamins, minerals and essential fatty acids.

**SERVES 1 CHILD**

1 ripe banana
¼ × 225 g (8 oz) pack silken (smooth) tofu
½ cup apple juice
1 tablespoon sunflower seeds
1 tablespoon flaxseed oil
½ level teaspoon lecithin granules

Liquidise all the ingredients to a smooth consistency and drink straight away. If left, the shake will continue to thicken because of the lecithin granules. (If you do leave it to thicken, it could always be served as a pudding.)

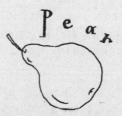

# Menu Ideas

## Sample menus for an 18-month-old

### MENU 1

**BREAKFAST**

Familia baby muesli with organic whole milk, soya milk,
or goat's milk
Wholemeal toast with Cashew Nut Butter (page 181)
Appropriate milk to drink

**LUNCH**

Salmon Fishcake (page 173), French beans and carrots
Banana Custard (page 189)
Water to drink

**TEA**

Beany Bake (page 153) and Salad Platter (page 158)
Fruit salad and live yogurt
Water to drink

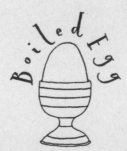

# MENU 2

### BREAKFAST
Kashi whole-grain cereal with banana, organic whole milk,
soya milk or goat's milk
Magical Muffin (page 201)
Appropriate milk to drink

### LUNCH
Liver Casserole (page 164), mashed potato and broccoli
Apple Crumble (page 194) and live yogurt
Water to drink

### TEA
Baked Eggs (page 156) and wholewheat toast
Fruit Smoothie (page 185)
Water to drink

# MENU 3

### BREAKFAST
Oat Porridge (page 106) with fresh fruit and organic whole
milk, soya milk or goat's milk
Rice cakes with Almond Butter (page 181)
Appropriate milk to drink

*continues* ▶

## LUNCH
Wholewheat spaghetti with Vegetable Rich Mince (page166)
Blueberry semolina (page 191)
Water to drink

## TEA
Potato Cakes (page 149) with salad and Salad Dressing
(page 156)
Pear pieces
Water to drink

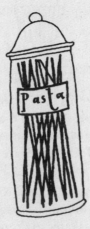

## Party menu

Wholemeal sandwiches (page 217)
Popcorn (page 205)
Plain corn chips or teddy bear crisps
Mini organic sausages
Magical Muffins (page 201)
Fresh Fruit Juice Jelly (page 192)
Date and Nut Truffles (page 203)
Almond Fruit Tarts (page 199) filled with 100 per cent fruit jam
Banana Birthday Cake (page 200)
Diluted apple and blackcurrant 100 per cent concentrate

## Ten-minute teas

Rice pasta spirals and frozen Quick and Easy Pasta Sauce
(page 136)
Pasta with Instant Fishy Pasta Sauce (page 174) and salad
Pasta with Walnut Pesto (page 137) and salad
Baked Eggs (page 156) and toast
Vegetable Frittata (page 154) and salad
Tofu Scramble (page 129) and toast
Grilled Sardine and Cheese Toasties (page 176) with cucumber,
celery and carrot sticks
Wholemeal sandwiches (see page 217)

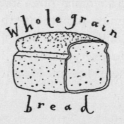

## Snack ideas

Mini rice cakes spread with nut or seed butters

Oat cakes spread with Hummus (see page 178) or
cottage cheese

Fruit slices: apple, pear, banana

100 per cent fruit and nut bars (e.g. sunflower bar by
Shepherd Boy)

Date Slice (page 202)

Shop-bought manna bread

An apple and a cube of Cheddar cheese

Sprouted nuts and seeds (be careful of choking –
see pages 38–40)

Carrot sticks and almond butter

Banana Birthday Cake (page 200)

Live natural yogurt, banana and wheatgerm

## Pizza Ideas

Believe it or not, pizzas can be healthy. You can now buy
wholemeal pizza bases from healthfood shops or, alternatively use wholemeal pitta breads, Oatcake Fingers (page
183) puzzled together to make a base or well-toasted wholemeal bread cut into a circular pizza shape.

Preparing pizzas is something that even the very
youngest in the family can do. Smooth on some tomato
sauce and chop up everything else and then let them
design their own. Here are some ideas for healthy toppings:

- Grated courgette
- Grated carrot
- Sliced mushrooms
- Sliced red, green and yellow peppers
- Grilled tuna chunks
- Chopped spinach
- Grated soya cheese, parmesan, mozzarella or crumbled goat's cheese
- Cooked chicken chunks
- Cooked salmon fillet
- Chopped parsley
- Thinly sliced red onion
- Cooked peas, broccoli florets or French beans

Place under a medium grill and cook for a few minutes until the edges are golden-brown and the cheese sizzling.

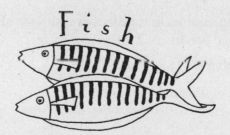

Fish

# Baked Potato Fillings

Baked potatoes are such a versatile food and most young-sters love them. By cooking the potatoes in their skins you retain many of the nutrients lost through other methods of cooking. Potatoes are rich in potassium, B vitamins and vitamin C, and are a wonderfully alkaline food. Further-more, a meal of baked potatoes is so quick and easy to prepare. You can also use other starchy vegetables as potato substitutes, such as sweet potato and yam.

- Hummus (page 178)

- Guacamole (page 179)

- Boston Baked Beans (page 155)

- Onion, mushroom and sweetcorn cooked in a little olive oil

- Bean Stew (page 142)

- Grated Cheddar cheese, goat's cheese or soya cheese with grated carrot and spring onion

- Tuna fish, cooked peas and sweetcorn with a little Salad Dressing (page 156)

- Mashed sardines in tomato sauce with freshly chopped parsley

- Vegetable Rich Mince (page 166)

- Tahini and mashed broccoli

- Mediterranean Ratatouille Bake (page 152)

- Diced chicken and red pepper with mayonnaise

- Mashed tofu

# Sandwich Fillings

Quick and easy teas are vital for hungry toddlers and children. Here are some nutritious ideas for a sandwich tea. Always use wholemeal bread or wholemeal pitta breads.

- Hummus (page 178) and cress

- Mashed hard-boiled egg and watercress

- Mashed sardines in tomato sauce

- Mashed hard-boiled egg and sardine (in oil)

- Marmite and cucumber

- Marmite and lettuce

- Cottage cheese and sweetcorn

- Grated cheese and grated apple

- Tuna and sweetcorn with a little Salad Dressing (page 156)

- Tuna mayonnaise and sliced cucumber

- Peanut butter and 100 per cent fruit raspberry jam

- Cashew butter and grated carrot

- Mashed banana and tahini

- Almond butter and molasses

- Walnut butter and chopped celery

- Iron Booster (page 117)

- Vegetable burger (shop-bought) and organic tomato ketchup

Serve with a large plate of chopped vegetables like carrot sticks, celery sticks, cucumber chunks, cauliflower florets, red pepper sticks and a handful of raisins in the middle. The nut butters (cashew, walnut, peanut and almond) can either be home-made (page181) or shop-bought.

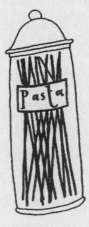

# Good Food–Healthy Children

As I HOPE I HAVE SHOWN, it is really very easy to feed your children a healthy diet, and the rewards far outweigh any extra effort involved. My children get ill, like any other children, but they are not debilitated by the odd cough or cold. Nor have they had antibiotics and I have no doubt that this is largely due to their diet.

If your children do get ill, here are some general tips to follow. The main point is to cut out the things that are known to hinder recovery. For example, dairy products of all sorts are highly mucus-forming and will only increase the length of a cold. Rice milk is an excellent substitute for cow's milk during acute illness and children love the taste as it is naturally sweet. It is also important to cut down on sugar, which suppresses the immune system. If your child seems a little off-colour on the day of a birthday party, think twice before sending him. The cakes, biscuits and fizzy drinks will undoubtedly make him feel worse. Feeding him lots of foods rich in vitamin C and zinc, on the other hand, will help to boost his immune system – along with plenty of fluids and rest. These simple changes can make a world of difference.

A child's vitality, strength and health can all be enhanced by diet. Feeding your child a fresh, wholesome and varied diet is the best possible start that you can give him. It is also the key to his future health.

# APPENDIX

# The Facts About Vitamins and Minerals

The following charts are for information only. Most children should get all the nutrients they require from a healthy, varied diet and a suitable multivitamin and mineral supplement per day (see Resources).

## Vitamins

### Fat-soluble vitamins

**Vitamin A (retinol and beta-carotene)**

Essential for growth, healthy skin and teeth, and protects against infection. It's also an antioxidant and immune-booster.

**Amount required (to prevent deficiency)**
Birth to 1 year: 350 mcgRE (1155 iu)
1–3 years: 400 mcgRE (1320 iu)
4–6 years 400 mcgRE (1320 iu)
(Note: RE = retinol equivalent; 1 mcgRE = 3.3 iu)

**Signs of deficiency**
Mouth ulcers, dry skin, poor hair condition, night blindness, increased susceptibility to infection, impaired growth.

## Vitamin D

Helps maintain strong and healthy bones by retaining calcium. Also supports tooth formation and muscle function.

**Amount required (to prevent deficiency)**
Birth–6 months: 8.5 mg
6 months–3 years: 7 mg
4+ yrs: 0 mg if exposed to sun

**Signs of deficiency**
Bone and tooth problems, rickets.

## Vitamin E

Aids in wound healing. Antioxidant which helps protect tissues from damage by pollutants. Good for the skin.

**Amount required (to prevent deficiency)**
Birth–1 year: 3 iu
1–3 years: 6 iu
4–6 years: 7 iu

**Signs of deficiency**
Dry skin, easy bruising, slow wound healing.

## Vitamin K

Essential for blood clotting.

**Amount required (to prevent deficiency)**
Birth–6 months: 5 mcg
6–12 months: 10 mcg
1–3 years: 15 mcg
4–6 years: 20 mcg

**Deficiency symptoms**
Haemorrhage (easy bleeding).

# Water-soluble vitamins

## Vitamin B1 (Thiamine)

Supports healthy functioning of the heart, muscles and nerves. Essential for energy production.

**Amount required (to prevent deficiency)**
Birth–1 year: 300 mcg
1–3 years: 500 mcg
4–6 years: 700 mcg

**Signs of deficiency**
Tiredness, memory loss, irritability, depression, prickly legs, stomach pains, constipation, tingling hands.

## Vitamin B2 (Riboflavin)

Helps turn fat, protein and carbohydrate into energy. Required to repair and maintain healthy skin, nails and eyes.

**Amount required (to prevent deficiency)**
Birth–12 months: 400 mcg
1–3 years: 600 mcg
4–6 years: 800 mcg

**Deficiency symptoms**
Light sensitivity, reddening of the eyes, dry skin, cracks at the corner of the mouth.

## Vitamin B3 (Niacin)

Essential for energy production, brain function and healthy skin.

**Amount required (to prevent deficiency)**
Birth–1 year: 6 mg
1–3 years: 8 mg
4–6 years: 11 mg

**Deficiency symptoms**
Lack of energy, irritability, insomnia, emotional instability, blood sugar fluctuations, headaches, eczema or dermatitis.

## Vitamin B5 (Pantothenic acid)

Essential for energy production. Involved in the production of adrenal and sex hormones. Maintains healthy hair and skin. Supports the sinuses.

**Amount required (to prevent deficiency)**
Birth–1 year: 3 mg
1–3 years: 4 mg
4–6 years: 4 mg

**Deficiency symptoms**
Lack of energy, teeth grinding, burning feet or tender heels, poor concentration.

## Vitamin B6 (Pyridoxine)

Involved in energy production. Essential for the healthy functioning of the nervous and digestive symptoms. Helps maintain healthy skin.

**Amount required (to prevent deficiency)**
Birth–1 year: 0.3–0.6 mg
1–3 years: 0.7 mg
4–6 years: 0.8 mg

**Deficiency symptoms**
Lack of energy, irritability, depression, flaky skin, tingling hands, muscle cramps or tremors.

## Vitamin B12 (Cobalamin)

Essential for energy production. Involved in growth and development, and the production of red blood cells. Helps the body use folic acid. Supports the healthy functioning of the nervous system.

**Amount required (to prevent deficiency)**
Birth–1 year: 0.3–0.5 mcg
1–3 years: 0.7 mcg
4–6 years: 0.9 mcg

**Deficiency symptoms**
Lack of energy, poor hair condition, constipation, irritability, loss of coordination.

## Biotin

Particularly important in childhood. Helps the body use essential fats. Assists in maintaining health of skin, hair, nerves and bone marrow.

**Amount required (to prevent deficiency)**
Birth–1 year: 10–15 mcg
1–3 years: 20 mcg
4–6 years: 25 mcg

**Deficiency symptoms**
Dry skin, poor hair condition, poor appetite or nausea, eczema or dermatitis, tender or sore muscles.

## Folic acid (folate)

Involved in growth, development and reproduction. Essential for brain and nerve function. Involved in production of red blood cells.

**Amount required (to prevent deficiency)**
Birth–1 year: 50 mcg
1–3 years: 70 mcg
4–6 years: 100 mcg

**Deficiency symptoms**
Anaemia, digestive problems, fatigue, cracked lips.

## Vitamin C

Strengthens the immune system and helps to fight infections. Supports wound healing. Important for the healthy growth of teeth, bones, gums, ligaments and blood vessels. Helps with the absorption of iron.

**Amount required (to prevent deficiency)**
Birth–1 year: 25 mg
1–3 years: 30 mg
4–6 years: 30 mg

**Deficiency symptoms**
Slow wound healing, bleeding gums, recurrent infections, allergies.

# Minerals

## Calcium

Plays a role in bone and tooth formation, blood clotting, heart rhythm, nerve transmission, muscle growth and contraction.

**Amount required (to prevent deficiency)**
Birth–1 year: 525 mg
1–3 years: 350 mg
4–6 years: 450 mg

**Deficiency symptoms**
Muscle cramps, irritability, insomnia, tooth decay.

## Magnesium

Needed for calcium metabolism. Strengthens bones and teeth and helps promote healthy muscles by acting as a muscle relaxant.

**Amount required (to prevent deficiency)**
Birth–6 months: 60 mg
6–12 months: 80 mg
1–3 years: 85 mg
4–6 years: 120 mg

**Deficiency symptoms**
Muscle tremors or spasms, insomnia, hyperactivity, constipation, fatigue, irritability, nervousness.

## Chromium

Involved in maintaining blood sugar levels and in the healthy functioning of the circulatory system.

**Amount required (to prevent deficiency)**
Birth–1 year: 10–60 mcg
1–3 years: 20–80 mcg
4–6 years: 30–120 mcg

**Deficiency symptoms**
Excessive or cold sweats, dizziness or irritability after six hours without food. Cold hands, excessive thirst, craving sweet foods, excessive drowsiness during the day.

## Iron

Supports growth and development in children. Involved in the production of haemoglobin. Helps build up resistance to disease.

**Amount required (to prevent deficiency)**
Birth–6 months: 4.3 mg
6–12 months: 7.8 mg
1–3 years: 6.9 mg
4–6 years: 6.1 mg

**Deficiency symptoms**
Fatigue, anaemia, pale skin, poor appetite, nausea, intolerance of the cold, intellectual impairment.

## Zinc

Promotes burn and wound healing, supports the immune system and builds resistance to disease. Involved in proper growth and development.

**Amount required (to prevent deficiency)**
Birth–6 months: 4 mg
6–12 months: 5 mg
1–3 years: 5 mg
4–6 years: 6.5 mg

**Deficiency symptoms**
White spots on fingernails, poor appetite, loss of taste and
smell, recurrent infections, poor growth.

## Selenium

Involved in the healthy functioning of cell membranes.
Stimulates the immune system to fight infections. Antioxidant
which protects the body against environmental pollutants.

**Amount required (to prevent deficiency)**
Birth–6 months: 10 mcg
6–12 months: 10 mcg
1–3 years: 15 mcg
4–6 years: 20 mcg

# Resources

## Children's vitamin and mineral supplements

Vitasorb liquid vitamins: Vitamin drops for babies from six months old (15 drops a day mixed with food). Available from Biocare Ltd, Lakeside, 180 Lifford Lane, King's Norton, Birmingham B30 3NT (Tel: 0121 433 3727).

Nutritec Vitaforte: Powdered multivitamins and minerals for toddlers from 12 months old (1 teaspoon a day added to food). Available from Biocare Ltd.

Bifidobacterium Infantis: Beneficial bacteria for bottle-fed babies (a quarter teaspoon added to food). Available from Biocare Ltd.

Flaxseed oil: Omega Nutrition Flaxseed Oil imported by Higher Nature, The Nutrition Centre, Burwash Common, East Sussex TN19 7LX (Tel: 01435 884668).

## Unhydrogenated margarines

Vitaquell and Vitaseig: Available at good healthfood stores; distributed by Brewhurst Health Food Supplies Ltd, Abbot Close, Oyster Lane, Byfleet, Surrey KT14 7JP
(Tel: 01932 354211).

## Marigold Swiss vegetable bouillon powder

Available at good supermarkets and healthfood shops, in original, low-salt and vegan versions. Distributed by Marigold Health Foods Ltd, 102 Camley Street, London NW1 0PF (Tel: 020 7388 4515).

## Breast-feeding counsellors

National Childbirth Trust, Alexandra House, Oldham Terrace, Acton, London W3 6NH (Tel: 0870 7703236). La Leche League, PO Box 29, West Bridgford, Nottingham, NG2 7NP (Tel: 0845 120 2918).

## Breast-feeding supplements

Health Plus Pregnancy Pack, designed for before, during and after pregnancy, available at good healthfood stores or direct from Health Plus Ltd, Dolphin House, 27 Craddle Hill Ind. Est., Seaford, East Sussex, BN25 3JE (Tel: 01323 872277).

Ante Natal Forte by Biocare, designed for before and during pregnancy and while breastfeeding, available from good healthfood stores or direct from Biocare Ltd (see page 230).

## Formula

Goat's Milk Infant Formula 'Nanny', available from good healthfood stores and chemists or direct from Vitacare Ltd, (Tel: 0800 328 5826).

## Organic food

The directory *Where to Buy Organic Food*, published by the Soil Association, contains details of farm shops, box delivery schemes and local retailers in your area. It costs £5 (inclusive of postage) or £4 to Soil Association members. The Soil Association can be contacted at Bristol House, 40–56 Victoria Street, Bristol, BS1 6BY (Tel: 0117 314 5000; Fax: 0117 314 5001; or E-mail: info@soilassociation.org).

Some firms now offer nationwide delivery to your door. One such company is Organics Direct (Tel: 020 7729 2828) or you can visit their web page: www.organics direct.co.uk

## Soya milks, desserts and tofu soya yogurts

Made by Provamel and available at good healthfood stores and supermarkets. Calcium-enriched soya milks for children over 12 months. All Provamel products are guaranteed to be free of genetically modified soya beans and they are committed to guaranteeing this 'for as long as is humanly possible'.

# Index